Nitric oxide in bone and joint disease

Nitric oxide research has emerged as one of the most important new areas in bone and joint diseases. This book is the first one to draw together current knowledge on the actions of this mediator and its role in such common diseases as arthritis and osteoporosis. It introduces the basic biology and biochemistry of nitric oxide, the immune responses and bone biology, and it reviews in depth the facts that we know today and the future promise of this exciting area of research. The book will give scientists and clinicians a unique insight and emphasizes potential new treatments that exploit our understanding of the role of nitric oxide in bone and joint disease.

The editors of this volume are all based at the internationally renowned Imperial College School of Medicine at the Hammersmith Campus in London. Their expertise and research activities span the full range from musculoskeletal research (Mika Hukkanen) to endocrine pathology (Julia Polak) through to orthopaedic surgery (Sean Hughes) and all have contributed numerous articles on regulatory factors and vascular function in disease states.

POSTGRADUATE MEDICAL SCIENCE

This important new series is based on the successful and internationally well-regarded specialist training programme at the Imperial College School of Medicine, Hammersmith Campus in London. Each volume provides an integrated and self-contained account of a key area of medical science, developed in conjunction with the course organizers and including contributions from specially invited authorities.

The aim of the series is to provide biomedical and clinical scientists with a reliable introduction to the theory and to the technical and clinical applications of each topic.

The volumes will be a valuable resource and guide for trainees in the medical and biomedical sciences and for laboratory-based scientists.

In the series:

Radiation protection of patients   R. Wootton

Image anaysis in histology: conventional and confocal microscopy   D. Springall, R. Wootton and J. Polak

Monoclonal antibodies   M. A. Ritter and H. M. Ladyman.

Molecular neuropathology   G. W. Roberts and J. M. Polak

Clinical gene analysis and manipulation   J. A. Z. Jankowski and J. M. Polak

Understanding cancer   M. Alison and C. Sarraf

Nitric oxide in bone and joint disease

BY

MIKA V. J. HUKKANEN, PhD
Lecturer in Histochemistry, Department of Histochemistry, Imperial College School of Medicine, London, UK

JULIA M. POLAK, PhD, FRCPath
Professor of Endocrine Pathology, Department of Histochemistry, Imperial College School of Medicine, London, UK

SEAN P. F. HUGHES, MS, FRCS
Professor of Orthopaedic Surgery, Department of Orthopaedic Surgery, Imperial College School of Medicine, London, UK

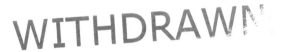

Published in association with
The Imperial College School of Medicine
University of London by

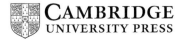 **CAMBRIDGE**
UNIVERSITY PRESS

PUBLISHED BY THE PRESS SYNDICATE OF THE UNIVERSITY OF CAMBRIDGE
The Pitt Building, Trumpington Street, Cambridge CB2 1RP, United Kingdom

CAMBRIDGE UNIVERSITY PRESS
The Edinburgh Building, Cambridge CB2 2RU, UK http://www.cup.cam.ac.uk
40 West 20th Street, New York, NY 10011-4211, USA http://www.cup.org
10 Stamford Road, Oakleigh, Melbourne 3166, Australia

First published 1998

Printed in the United Kingdom at the University Press, Cambridge

Typeset in Times 10/13pt [KT]

A catalogue record for this book is available from the British Library

Library of Congress Cataloguing in Publication data

Nitric oxide in bone and joint disease / [edited] by Mika V. J. Hukkanen, Julia M. Polak, Sean P. F.
Hughes.
    p.   cm. – (Postgraduate medical science)
"Published in association with the Imperial College School of Medicine, University of London."
Includes bibliographical references and index.
ISBN 0 521 59220 8 (hardback)
1. Bones – Diseases – Pathophysiology.   2. Joints – Diseases – Pathophysiology.   3. Nitric oxide –
Pathophysiology.   I. Hukkanen, Mika V. J., 1962– .   II. Polak, Julia M.   III. Hughes, Sean.
IV. Imperial College School of Medicine. V. Series.
[DNLM: 1. Bone Diseases – immunology.   2. Joint Diseases – immunology.   3. Nitric Oxide –
physiology.   4. Bone and Bones – metabolism.   WE 225 N731 1998]
RC930.4.N56 1998
616.7'107–dc21   98-14672 CIP
DNLM/DLC
for Library of Congress

ISBN 0 521 59220   8 hardback

Contents

Contributors

David R. Blake   Department of Postgraduate Medicine, University of Bath, Claverton Downs, Bath BA2 7AI, UK

Lee D. K. Buttery   Department of Histochemistry, Division of Diagnostic and Investigative Sciences, Imperial College School of Medicine, Hammersmith Campus, Du Cane Road, London W12 0NN, UK

Min Cao   Department of Orthopaedic Surgery, University of Pittsburgh School of Medicine, Pittsburgh, PA 15261, USA

Tim J. Chambers   Department of Histopathology, St George's Hospital Medical School, London SW17 0RE, UK

Jade W. M. Chow   Department of Histopathology, St. George's Hospital Medical School, London SW17 0RE, UK

Steven A. Corbett   Departments of Orthopaedics and Histochemistry, Imperial College School of Medicine, Hammersmith Campus, Du Cane Road, London W12 0NN, UK

Peter Croucher   Department of Human Metabolism and Clinical Biochemistry, University of Sheffield Medical School, Sheffield S10 2RX, UK

Christopher H. Evans   Departments of Orthopaedic Surgery and Molecular Genetics, University of Pittsburgh School of Medicine, Pittsburgh, PA 15261, USA

William R. Ferrell   Institute of Biomedical and Life Sciences, University of Glasgow, Glasgow G12 8QQ, UK

Simon Fox   Department of Histopathology, St George's Hospital Medical School, London SW17 0RE, UK

John A. Frangos	Department of Bioengineering, University of California, San Diego, La Jolla, CA 92093-0412, USA
Hans-Jorg Häuselmann	Department of Rheumatology, University of Zurich, CH 8091, Switzerland
Yukio Hirata	Second Department of Internal Medicine, Tokyo Medical and Dental University, 1-5-45, Yushima, Bunkyo-ku, Tokyo, Japan
Ron L. Howard	Department of Medical Physics, Atkinson Morley's Hospital, London, SW20 0NE, UK
Francis J. Hughes	Department of Periodontology, St Bartholomews and Royal London School of Medicine and Dentistry, London E1 2AD, UK
Sean P. F. Hughes	Department of Orthopaedic Surgery, Imperial College School of Medicine, Hammersmith Campus, Du Cane Road, London W12 0NN, UK
Mika V. J. Hukkanen	Department of Histochemistry, Division of Diagnostic and Investigative Sciences, Imperial College School of Medicine, Hammersmith Campus, Du Cane Road, London W12 0NN, UK
Christopher J. Jagger	Department of Histopathology, St. George's Hospital Medical School, London SW17 0RE, UK
Janos M. Kanczler	Department of Postgraduate Medicine, University of Bath, Claverton Downs, Bath BA2 7AI, UK
Lance E. Lanyon	Department of Veterinary Basic Sciences, The Royal Veterinary College, London NW1 0TU, UK
Jenny M. Lean	Department of Histopathology, St George's Hospital Medical School, London SW17 0RE, UK
Foo Y. Liew	Department of Immunology and Centre for Rheumatic Diseases, University of Glasgow, Glasgow G11 6NT, UK
John C. Lockhart	Institute of Biomedical and Life Sciences, University of Glasgow, Glasgow G12 8QQ, UK
Iain MacIntyre	The William Harvey Research Institute, Charterhouse Square, London EC1M 6BQ, UK
Lucia Mancini	The William Harvey Research Institute, Charterhouse Square, London EC1M 6BQ, UK
Todd N. McAllister	Department of Bioengineering, University of California, San Diego, La Jolla, CA 92093-0412, USA

Ian D. McCarthy   Department of Orthopaedic Surgery, Imperial College School of
                            Medicine, Hammersmith Campus, Du Cane Road, London W12 0NN,
                            UK

Iain B. McInnes   Department of Immunology and Centre for Rheumatic Diseases,
                            University of Glasgow, Glasgow G11 6NT, UK

Lorraine McMurdo   Institute of Biomedical and Life Sciences, University of Glasgow,
                            Glasgow G12 8QQ, UK

Frederick T. Mitchell   Department of Medical Physics, St George's Hospital Medical School,
                            London, SW17 0QT, UK

Nobuyuki Miyasaka   First Department of Internal Medicine, Tokyo Medical and Dental
                            University, 1-5-45, Yushima, Bunkyo-ku, Tokyo, Japan

Salvador Moncada   Cruciform Project for Strategic Medical Research, University College
                            London, London WC1E 6JJ, UK

Niloufar   The William Harvey Research Institute, Charterhouse Square, London
Moradi-Bidhendi   EC1M 6BQ, UK

Babatunde Oyajobi   Department of Human Metabolism and Clinical Biochemistry,
                            University of Sheffield Medical School, Sheffield S10 2RX, UK

Andrew A. Pitsillides   Department of Veterinary Basic Sciences, The Royal Veterinary
                            College, London NW1 0TU, UK

Julia M. Polak   Department of Histochemistry, Division of Diagnostic and
                            Investigative Sciences, Imperial College School of Medicine,
                            Hammersmith Campus, Du Cane Road, London W12 0NN, UK

Shamim Rahman   Department of Human Metabolism and Clinical Biochemistry,
                            University of Sheffield Medical School, Sheffield S10 2RX, UK

Stuart H. Ralston   Bone Research Group, Department of Medicine and Therapeutics,
                            University of Aberdeen Medical School, Aberdeen AB9 2ZD, UK

Michael Rogers   Department of Human Metabolism and Clinical Biochemistry,
                            University of Sheffield Medical School, Sheffield S10 2RX, UK

R. Graham G. Russell   Department of Human Metabolism and Clinical Biochemistry,
                            University of Sheffield Medical School, Sheffield S10 2RX, UK

Tulin Sahinoglu   Department of Postgraduate Medicine, University of Bath, Claverton
                            Downs, Bath BA2 7AI, UK

Daniela Salvemini   Discovery Pharmacology, G.D. Searle Co., St Louis, MO 63167, USA

Andrew Scutt   Department of Human Metabolism and Clinical Biochemistry, University of Sheffield Medical School, Sheffield S10 2RX, UK

Rolf Smalt   Department of Histopathology, St George's Hospital Medical School, London SW17 0RE, UK

Maja Stefanovic-Racic   Department of Orthopaedic Surgery, University of Pittsburgh School of Medicine, Pittsburgh, PA 15261, USA

Cliff R. Stevens   Department of Postgraduate Medicine, Bath University, Claverton Downs, Bath BA2 7AI, UK

Patrick Vallance   Cruciform Project for Strategic Medical Research, University College London, London WC1E 6JJ, UK

Preface

What is formed for long duration arrives slowly to its maturity
Samuel Johnson, *The Rambler* (1750–52), p. 169.

Nitric oxide was considered for a long time to be a harmful gas produced in toxic car fumes. We now know that nitric oxide is actually provided in abundance by our bodies and a remarkable field has burgeoned: 'the nitric oxide field'. Nitric oxide is a powerful modulator of bodily function and many books, monographs and treatises have been published that describe its production by and actions on specific organ systems, including the cardiovascular, respiratory and gastrointestinal systems. This book, however, is unique and no other, to our knowledge, has been published which deals with the subject of nitric oxide in bone and joint disease. This is the culmination of intense research into the release of nitric oxide and its effects on osteoblasts, osteoclasts and many other bone cells as well as its involvement in bone destruction and remodelling.

The first section of the book gives a masterly overview of the nitric oxide field by Moncada and Vallance and deals principally with the biology and pathophysiology of nitric oxide. This section also deals with nitric oxide responses in immunological processes and to proinflammatory cytokines involved in bone disease. The second section deals with inflammation (arthritides) and demonstrates the role of nitric oxide in experimental models of arthritis using specific inhibitors and its role in human arthritides. The interactions of prostaglandins and/or nitric oxide in the control of blood flow and cartilage matrix turnover and the interactions of nitric oxide with reactive oxygen species are also dealt with in detail. Section three deals specifically with the expression and functions of nitric oxide in different cell types. Blood flow, fluid stress, mechanical strain and their influence on human pathology are all discussed in Section four.

On behalf of my co-editors, I would like to express our gratitude to all the experts, and the book has a fabulous constellation of them, who set aside time for the preparation of their respective impressive contributions. I can think of no more fitting way to celebrate the anniversary of my transplant than with the publication of this distinguished volume.

Many thanks

Julia M. Polak
London

Nitric oxide and cytokines – an introduction

1

A brief overview of the biology of nitric oxide

PATRICK VALLANCE and SALVADOR MONCADA

1.1 Introduction

Nitric oxide (NO) is an inorganic gas; it is a paramagnetic species that has an unpaired electron in its outer orbit, a free radical. In 1987, the suggestion that this small and potentially toxic molecule might act as a biological mediator (Palmer, Ferrige and Moncada, 1987) was met with surprise and scepticism. However, ten years later there are over 13 000 publications on NO and important biological roles have been identified in the cardiovascular, respiratory, nervous, genitourinary, gastrointestinal, host defence, haemopoietic and musculoskeletal systems (for review, see Moncada and Higgs, 1995).

1.2 Synthesis of NO

Nitric oxide is synthesized from L-arginine by the action of nitric oxide synthase (NOS). The nitrogen is derived from one of the guanidino nitrogens of arginine; the oxygen comes from molecular oxygen (Figure 1.1). The amino acid L-citrulline is formed as a by-product of the reaction.

Three isoforms of NOS have been identified: an endothelial isoform (eNOS), a neuronal isoform (nNOS) and an isoform induced by immunological or inflammatory stimuli (iNOS). The genes encoding these isoforms are located on human chromosome 7 (eNOS), 12 (nNOS) and 17 (iNOS). The NOSs are haemoproteins that have oxidative and reductive domains and catalyse the 5-electron reduction of arginine to NO. They share homology with cytochrome P450 reductases and have binding sites for NADPH, flavoproteins, biopterin and calmodulin (Figure 1.2). Calmodulin is required for the electron flow from NADPH to the reductase domain of the enzyme and from the reductase domain to the haem group. Calmodulin may act as a molecular switch, inducing a conformational change in NOS that facilitates transfer of electrons. Calmodulin binds rapidly and reversibly to eNOS and nNOS; binding triggers a high rate of electron transfer to the haem moiety. In contrast, calmodulin is bound tightly to iNOS, and this provides a continuously available, but suboptimal, means of haem reduction that is only increased substantially on binding of L-arginine. Substrate control of haem reduction makes iNOS more similar to

3

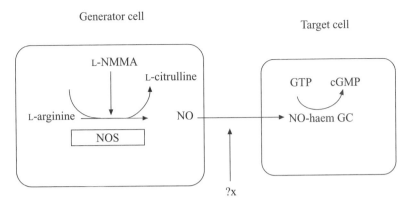

Figure 1.1. NOS catalyses the synthesis of NO from L-arginine and molecular oxygen; L-citrulline is the by-product. NO itself might inhibit the activity of NOS by interacting with the haem moiety of this enzyme. Physiological effects are produced after NO binds to the haem moiety of guanylyl cyclase and activates this enzyme to product cGMP from GTP in target and generator cells. Molecules (x) that stabilize NO have been proposed. NO is also vulnerable to inactivation by other radicals.

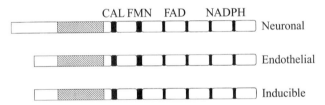

Figure 1.2. The gene for neuronal NOS is located on chromosome 12, for the endothelial enzyme on chromosome 7 and for the inducible enzyme on chromosome 17. Overall homology is around 50%. Shaded area represents putative arginine-binding site.

cytochrome P450. One important consequence of the differences between the isoforms is that the overall activity of eNOS and nNOS is dependent on the prevailing concentration of calcium/calmodulin whereas iNOS activity is often functionally independent of calcium concentration. Intriguingly, iNOS isolated from rabbit chondrocytes does not have calmodulin bound tightly and its activity is calcium/calmodulin-dependent (Palmer *et al.*, 1993). The reasons for this are not known, and it remains to be determined whether post-translational modifications of iNOS or differences in regulation of calmodulin may lead to the induction of calcium/calmodulin-dependent iNOS in other cells or tissues.

1.3 Expression of NOS isoforms

eNOS and nNOS are constitutive enzymes, expressed in a variety of cell types. eNOS has been identified in endothelial cells, endocardial cells, platelets, epithelial cells and certain white cells. nNOS is located primarily in neurones but is also expressed in skeletal muscle (Kobzik *et al.*, 1994). Although these enzymes are expressed constitutively, it is clear that further expression may be induced; for example oestrogens increase expression of eNOS in endothelial cells and of nNOS in the brain (Weiner *et al.*, 1994). Expression can also be down-regulated; certain cytokines (e.g. tumour necrosis factor (TNF) α) decrease expression of eNOS in endothelial cells, at least in some experimental models.

Expression of iNOS is induced by exposure of cells to bacterial endotoxin or certain proinflammatory cytokines, including interleukin-1β (IL-1β), TNFα and interferon γ (IFN-γ) (for review, see Wong and Billiar (1995)). iNOS can be induced in a wide variety of cells including macrophages, vascular smooth muscle and endothelial cells, cardiac myocytes, hepatocytes, Küppfer cells, glial cells and osteoblasts and osteoclast-like cells (Brandi *et al.*, 1995; Hukkanen *et al.*, 1995). Induction of iNOS forms a major part of 'non-specific' immunity (Chapter 2). Until recently, it was thought that iNOS was not expressed constitutively; however, there is now evidence that constitutive expression of iNOS may also occur (Chapter 2). The significance of this observation remains to be determined.

1.4 Targets for NO

Soluble guanylyl cyclase appears to be the major target enzyme for NO generated as part of normal physiology (Figure 1.1). The NO binds to the haem moiety of guanylyl cyclase and this activates the enzyme to generate cyclic GMP (cGMP) from GTP. cGMP has a wide variety of effects in different target cells and these have been reviewed extensively elsewhere (McDonald and Murad, 1996). It is not known whether there is a single soluble guanylyl cyclase or whether different tissues express different isoforms. Recently, a specific inhibitor of guanylyl cyclase has been developed (Garthwaite *et al.*, 1995) and use of this compound confirms that many of the physiological actions of the L-arginine: NO pathway can be fully accounted for by activation of guanylyl cyclase.

NO is a radical that interacts with haem groups and other moieties that contain transition metals. Therefore, there is the potential for NO to interact with any haem-containing enzyme and any of the vast range of enzymes that rely on transition metals for activity. Although many such interactions have been described, their physiological significance is uncertain. However, the interactions between NO and cytochrome *c* oxidase are of particular interest. NO causes reversible inhibition of cytochrome *c* oxidase and might thereby exert a continuous brake on oxygen consumption (Cleeter *et al.*, 1994). In contrast, peroxynitrite (ONOO$^-$), a product of the reaction between NO and the superoxide anion (O$_2^-$), irreversibly inhibits complexes I and III of the respiratory cycle and this might lead to significant impairment of oxidative respiration under conditions of inflammation or systemic infection, in which iNOS is expressed and O$_2^-$ generation is increased (Lizasoain *et al.*, 1996).

1.5 NO transport

NOSs generate free NO, and guanylyl cyclase responds to free NO. However, NO may react with other species, and various adducts of NO have been proposed as carriers or stabilizing molecules. Interest has focused on nitrosothiols, including nitrosoglutathione (Upchurch, Welch and Loscalzo, 1995). While it is still unclear whether this compound subserves any physiological function, it has a profile of activity that differs from other NO donors, including glyceryl trinitrate and sodium nitroprusside, in that nitrosoglutathione has prominent anti-platelet effects at concentrations that barely alter vascular tone (Radomski *et al.*, 1992; de Belder *et al.*, 1994). This observation raises the possibility that NO donors with tissue specificity may be developed. Recently, it has also been suggested that haemoglobin may act as a carrier molecule for NO (Jia, Bonaventura and Stamler, 1996). This suggestion is based upon the chemical detection of products of the interactions between haemoglobin and NO; however, there is no evidence yet for any functional significance of such interactions other than as a mechanism to deactivate free NO.

1.6 Conclusions

The L-arginine:NO pathway is a highly conserved pathway throughout evolution for inter- and intracellular signalling. Constitutively expressed NOSs are involved in a variety of physiological functions whereas the inducible isoform is part of the immune response. As selective inhibitors of each isoform become available, and with the advent of 'knockout' mice lacking the ability to express individual isoforms, the roles of NO in physiology and pathophysiology are gradually becoming clearer.

References

Brandi, M. L., Hukkanen, M., Umeda, T. *et al.* (1995) Bidirectional regulation of osteoclast function by nitric oxide synthase isoforms. *Proc. Natl. Acad. Sci., USA* **92**, 2954–2958.

Cleeter, M. W., Cooper, J. M., Darley-Usmar, V. M., Moncada, S. and Schapira, A. H. (1994) Reversible inhibition of cytochrome *c* oxidase, the terminal enzyme of the mitochondrial respiratory chain, by nitric oxide. Implications for neurodegenerative diseases. *FEBS Lett.* **345**: 50–54.

de Belder, A. J., MacAllister, R., Radomski, M. W., Moncada, S. and Vallance, P. (1994) Effects of *S*-nitroso-glutathione in the human forearm circulation: evidence for selective inhibition of platelet activation. *Cardiovasc. Res.* **28**, 691–694.

Garthwaite, J., Southam, E., Boulton, C. L., Nielsen, E. B., Schmidt, K. and Mayer, B. (1995) Potent and selective inhibition of nitric oxide-sensitive guanylyl cyclase by 1*H*-(1,2,4)-oxadiazolo-(4,3-a)-quinoxalin-1-one. *Mol. Pharmacol.* **48**, 184–188.

Hukkanen, M., Hughes, F. J., Buttery, L. D. *et al.* (1995) Cytokine-stimulated expression of inducible nitric oxide synthase by mouse, rat and human osteoplast-like cells and its functional role in osteoblast metabolic activity. *Endocrinology* **136**, 5445–5453.

Jia, L., Bonaventura, J. and Stamler, J. S. (1996) *S*-Nitrosohaemoglobin: a dynamic activity of blood involved in vascular control. *Nature* **380**, 221–226.

Kobzik, L., Reid, M. B., Bredt, D. S. and Stamler, J. S. (1994) Nitric oxide in skeletal muscle. *Nature* **372**, 546–548.

Lizasoain, I., Moro, M. A., Knowles, R. G., Darley-Usmar, V. and Moncada, S. (1996) Nitric oxide and peroxynitrite exert distinct effects on mitochondrial respiration which are differentially blocked by glutathione or glucose. *Biochem. J.* **314**, 877–880.

McDonald, L. J. and Murad, F. (1996) Nitric oxide and cyclic GMP signaling. *Proc. Soc. Exp. Biol. Med.* **211**, 1–6.

Moncada, S. and Higgs, E. A. (1995) Molecular mechanisms and therapeutic strategies related to nitric oxide. *FASEB J.* **9**, 1319–1330.

Palmer, R. M., Ferrige, A. G. and Moncada, S. (1987) Nitric oxide release accounts for the biological activity of endothelium-derived relaxing factor. *Nature* **327**, 524–526.

Palmer, R. M., Hickery, M. S., Charles, I.G., Moncada, S. and Bayliss, M. T. (1993) Induction of nitric oxide synthase in human chondrocytes. *Biochem. Biophys. Res. Commun.* **193**, 398–405.

Radomski, M. W., Rees, D. D., Dutra, A. and Moncada, S. (1992) *S*-Nitroso-glutathione inhibits platelet activation *in vitro* and *in vivo*. *Br. J. Pharmacol.* **107**, 745–749.

Upchurch, G. R. Jr, Welch, G. N. and Loscalzo, J. (1995) *S*-Nitrosothiols: chemistry, biochemistry and biological actions. *Adv. Pharmacol.* **34**, 343–349.

Weiner, C. P., Lizasoain, I., Baylis, S. A., Knowles, R. G., Charles, I. G. and Moncada, S. (1994) Induction of calcium-dependent nitric oxide synthases by sex hormones. *Proc. Natl. Acad. Sci., USA* **91**, 5212–5216.

Wong, J. M. and Billiar, T. R. (1995) Regulation and function of inducible nitric oxide synthase during sepsis and acute inflammation. *Adv. Pharmacol.* **34**, 155–170.

2

Nitric oxide and immune responses

IAIN B. MCINNES and FOO Y. LIEW

2.1 Introduction

In 1987, NO was recognised as the previously elusive endothelium-derived relaxing factor (Ignarro et al., 1987; Palmer, Ferrige and Moncada, 1987). Subsequently, NO emerged as a key regulatory molecule in numerous and diverse physiological and pathophysiological processes. This chapter will review the role of NO in the effector phase and the regulation of immune responses.

2.2 NOS isoforms

NO is generated by the NOS isoforms, which catalyse the conversion of L-arginine to L-citrulline. Three isoforms have been identified and their enzymology extensively studied (Chapter 1; Bredt and Snyder, 1994; Nathan and Xie, 1994). Endothelial and neuronal NOS are constitutively expressed and are capable of rapid onset, short-lived generation of low concentrations of NO (together termed cNOS). In contrast, iNOS is present in cells only after specific up-regulation. NOS isoforms share 30–40% homology with cytochrome P450 reductase (CPR), with consensus sequences for redox-active cofactors including NADPH, FAD and FMN. In contrast, expression of iNOS requires novel protein synthesis and thereafter generates high concentrations of NO over prolonged periods. As with cNOS, iNOS forms dimers in the presence of tetrahydrobiopterin (BH$_4$), haem and L-arginine. However, calmodulin is tightly bound to a basic, hydrophobic site on iNOS, and enzyme activity is independent of ambient calcium concentration (Cho et al., 1992). iNOS was first cloned from murine macrophages and subsequently from human hepatocytes and chondrocytes (Cho et al., 1992; Charles et al., 1993; Geller et al., 1993; Bredt and Snyder, 1994; Nathan and Xie, 1994). Human iNOS shares 50–60% homology with human cNOS and 80% with murine iNOS and is located on chromosome 17. Widespread tissue distribution of iNOS has been reported, with expression observed in human keratinocytes, hepatocytes, osteoblasts/osteoclasts, chondrocytes, uterine smooth muscle cells, mesangial cells, dermal fibroblasts, neutrophils and respiratory epithelial cells (Nathan and Xie, 1994). Expression in human tumours has also been observed, including colorectal adenocarcinoma and glioblastoma. However, considerable controversy surrounds the presence and activity of iNOS in human macrophages. Whereas some authors have demonstrated NO production directly, or L-arginine-/NO-dependent activity (Denis, 1991; Zembala *et al.*, 1994; Burkrinsky *et al.*, 1995; Dugas *et al.*, 1995), others have been unable to detect any evidence of iNOS activity at all (Schneemann *et al.*, 1993). The required stimuli for iNOS up-regulation in human macrophages appear to differ from those in rodents, and where NO production has been detected, it is of an order of magnitude lower than that observed in rodent macrophages. Whether this represents a functionally significant difference in the precise role of NO in the generation of immune responses in rodents compared with humans remains unclear. Nevertheless, the widespread tissue distribution of iNOS confers upon host tissue cells of either species the ability to contribute to immune responses through high output NO generation.

2.3 Regulation of NOS during immune responses

Modulation of immune responses requires rapid elaboration of immunoactive mediators. Since NO may not be stored in 'bioactive' form, its concentration in tissues and, therefore, its contribution to immunity is regulated through NOS activity. cNOS generates NO at picomolar concentrations in response to local vasoactive mediators (such as bradykinin, thrombin, histamine, acetylcholine or 5-hydroxytryptamine), to cytokines (e.g. IL-1β, endothelin-3) or to physical factors (including increased blood flow or shear stress) (reviewed in Chapters 13 and 14). Whether cNOS output may be further up-regulated is unclear. Evidence for induction of a novel isoform resembling 'nNOS' by IL-1β and lipopolysaccharide (LPS) in chondrocytes from osteoarthritic patients has been reported, indicating that the delineation between low and high output NOS on the basis of calcium dependency alone may be oversimplified (Amin *et al.*, 1995).

The predominant source of NO in inflammatory lesions, however, is iNOS. Given the ubiquitous effects of NO in inflammatory lesions, it might be anticipated that many facors will control iNOS expression and activity. iNOS may be activated *in vitro* by cytokines, microbial products (particularly LPS and superantigen toxins), picolinic acid, cAMP-elevating agents and physical factors, including UV light or trauma (Nathan and Xie, 1994; Lyons, 1995). Cytokines appear to exert the major regulatory influence *in vivo*. IFN-γ is a potent inducer of NO production by rodent macrophages and endothelial cells, in synergy with LPS (Liew and Cox, 1991). IL-1β and TNFα also increase iNOS expression in many cells, either alone or in synergistic combination (Liew, 1994). Cytokine requirements vary with the species and tissue origin of cells. For example, rodent smooth muscle cells respond to IL-1β either alone or in synergy with IFN-γ or TNFα, whereas human vascular smooth muscle cells require a combination of LPS, IFN-γ and TNFα for NO production. Similarly, rodent hepatocytes respond to LPS alone, whereas human hepatocytes require a combination of LPS, IFN-γ, TNFα and IL-2 (Geller *et al.*, 1993; Liew, 1994; Nathan and Xie, 1994; Lyons, 1995).

The multiplicity of activating factors is matched by a wide range of inhibitory agents. TGFβ, IL-4, IL-8, IL-10 (indirectly through effects on TNFα production), IL-13, macrophage inflammatory protein 1α (MIP-1α), epidermal growth factor (EGF), platelet-derived growth factor (PDGF), and fibroblast growth factor (FGF) all oppose iNOS activation (Liew, 1994; Nathan and Xie, 1994; Lyons, 1995). Again species and tissue specificity appear crucial. TGFβ inhibits rodent macrophage and endothelial iNOS expression but enhances NO production in Swiss 3T3 fibroblasts (Gilbert and Herschman, 1993). Moreover, IL-10 has been shown to increase iNOS activity in avian osteoclasts (Sunyer et al., 1996), as has IL-4 in human macrophages (Dugas et al., 1995). The temporal sequence of ligand binding appears important, since pre-exposure of macrophages to LPS suppresses subsequent IFN-γ-induced NO production. Such observations emphasize the difficulties attached to extrapolation between species and cell types. Furthermore, it has only recently been appreciated that iNOS may be 'constitutively' present in human tissues such as lung, retina, skeletal muscle or CNS in the absence of specific up-regulatory factors (Nathan and Xie, 1994). This suggests that, in addition to a postulated responsive role in inflammation, iNOS may also be involved in normal physiological regulation.

Engagement of class II MHC either by allo-specific monoclonal antibodies or by bacterial superantigens (staphylococcal enterotoxin B (SEB), toxic shock syndrome toxin 1 (TSST-1)) in the presence of syngeneic lymphocytes increases NO production by macrophages (Isobe and Nakashima, 1992; Tao and Stout, 1993). The requirement for T cells in this model can be replaced by addition of exogenous IFN-γ (I. B. McInnes, unpublished observations). Similarly, activation of macrophage NO synthesis follows crosslinking of CD69 by antibody. Cell–cell contact between T lymphocytes of both T_H1 and T_H2 subsets and macrophages leads to iNOS expression mediated in part through CD40/CD40 ligand and LFA-1/ICAM-1 (lymphocyte function-associated antigen 1/intercellular adhesion molecule 1). Thus, homo- or heterotypic cell contact can induce NO synthesis in an inflammatory lesion. The relative contribution of such mechanisms in the context of high levels of cytokine production is currently unclear.

These diverse factors mediate regulation at multiple levels. Two promoter/enhancer sites are found 5' to the murine iNOS gene (Bredt and Snyder, 1994; Nathan and Xie, 1994). Region 1 (-50 to -200 bp) contains LPS-responsive elements containing binding sites for the nuclear factors activator protein 1 (AP-1), NF-IL6 and NF-κB, whereas region 2 (~ 1000 bp upstream) contains an interferon-specific response element (IRE). Macrophages from IFN-γ-related transcription factor-1 (IRF-1) knockout mice do not produce NO in response to IFN-γ, confirming a role for IRF-1 in regulating iNOS expression, mediated partly through enhancement of LPS-dependent effects (Kamijo et al., 1994). A hypoxia-responsive enhancer has recently been identified (-209 to -207 bp) (Mellilo et al., 1995), indicating that other factors can facilitate iNOS transcription in addition to cytokine-dependent elements. Transcriptional regulation of the human iNOS gene is more complex. Involvement of a NF-κB binding site (-106 to -115 bp) has been demonstrated using mutant constructs of vascular smooth muscle iNOS (Kolyada, Savikovsky and Madias, 1996) and recent studies of hepatocyte iNOS responsiveness to IL-1β, TNFα and IFN-γ revealed three cytokine responsive elements -3.8 to -16 kb upstream from the iNOS gene (de Vera *et al.*, 1996). This is in contrast to the shorter regulatory 5' region ($\sim$ 1 kb) of rodent iNOS. Further characterization of the iNOS promoter sites will elucidate interspecies differences currently detected at the protein expression and functional level, particularly in comparison of rodent and human macrophage activation.

Post-transcriptional modification of mRNA by many regulatory factors is reported, but it is unclear at present whether these effects are directly mediated on mRNA stability or at earlier or later stages. Therefore, mRNA stability is increased by IFN-γ and reduced by TNFα, TGFβ and IL-4 in murine macrophages (Nathan and Xie, 1994). Post-translational regulation also occurs. cNOS is calcium and calmodulin dependent, whereas iNOS requires only the physiological concentrations of calcium present in resting cells, and as such is resistant to calmodulin antagonists (Cho *et al.*, 1992; Bredt and Snyder, 1994; Nathan and Xie, 1994). NOS activity may also be modified by phosphorylation. eNOS and nNOS share consensus sequences for cAMP-dependent protein kinase phosphorylation (Bredt and Snyder, 1994). Protein kinase C, cGMP-dependent kinase and calcium/calmodulin-dependent kinase have also been implicated in cNOS phosphorylation, raising the possibility of regulatory feedback loops whereby the reaction of NO with target enzymes may increase kinase activity, with consequent suppression of NOS activity (Bredt and Snyder, 1994). However, whether significant phosphorylation occurs *in vivo* to modify directly enzymatic activity, cofactor function or iNOS compartmentalization is unclear. Finally, haem-binding proteins are subject to down-regulation by NO. Therefore, direct inhibition of NOS activity by NO itself has been reported (Assreuy *et al.*, 1993). Substrate availability *in vitro* is determined by the relative presence of L-arginine, which itself is dependent on argininosuccinate synthetase, which converts L-citrulline to L-arginine, and on arginase in macrophages. Similarly, cofactor availability is critical. IFN-γ induces the enzyme GTP cyclohydroxylase I, which is the rate-limiting enzyme in the biopterin synthesis pathway responsible for the generation of tetrahydrobiopterin. Although the latter is depleted after long-term culture of human endothelial cells or fibroblasts, it is unclear whether this represents an *in vitro* artefact, or an *in vivo* example of coordinate function by IFN-γ.

Glucocorticoids, which are potent immunosuppressive agents *in vivo*, inhibit iNOS-dependent activity. (Di Rosa *et al.*, 1990). The rate of iNOS transcription is reduced, and although mRNA is briefly stabilized, translation is significantly retarded and degradation of iNOS protein is enhanced (Kunz *et al.*, 1996). NF-κB p50 or p65 nuclear translocation is unaffected, but NF-κB and not AP-1 binding in the iNOS promoter region is prevented (Kleinert *et al.*, 1996). L-N^{ω}-substituted arginines also inhibit NOS activity in biological systems. L-N^{ω}-Methylarginine (L-NMMA) is commonly used when no isoform specificity is necessary. No isoform specific inhibitor has yet been identified, although L-N^{ω}-nitroarginine

(L-NNA) exhibits relative specificity for cNOS as does L-N^ω-aminoarginine for iNOS. Aminoguanidine and N-iminoethyl-L-lysine (L-NIL) are further 'iNOS selective' inhibitors often used in animal models. However, mice in which the eNOS, nNOS and iNOS genes, respectively, have been specifically targeted have now been generated, allowing definitive investigation of the specific contribution of individual isoforms to be evaluated in different biological systems *in vivo* (Huang *et al.*, 1995; MacMicking *et al.*, 1995; Wei *et al.*, 1995).

2.4 NO in early inflammation

The extensive tissue distribution and wide range of potential regulatory factors clearly indicate roles for NO at multiple levels in host defence. Such effects may be demonstrated in both innate and antigen-specific immune responses. By virtue of its endothelium-derived relaxation factor (EDRF) activity, NO can induce vasodilatation through relaxation of vascular smooth muscle, leading to erythema and increased local temperature (Chapter 4; for review, see Schmidt and Walter (1994)). Data from murine dextran- and carrageenan-induced models of inflammation indicate that NO also induces clinically detectable oedema formation through alteration of endothelial permeability. Therefore, two features of the classical inflammatory response are regulated by NO. A further level of complexity lies in the interaction of iNOS with constitutive and inducible isoforms of cyclooxygenase and their product, the prostaglandins.

NO inhibits platelet aggregation as a function of its cardioprotective role, through production of cGMP (Schmidt and Walter, 1994). Subsequent studies of ischaemia–reperfusion in mesenteric vessels and myocardium have indicated that NO also reduces neutrophil adhesion through pathways dependent on CD11/CD18, ICAM-1 and P-selectin and by scavenging reactive oxygen intermediates, which enhance adhesion (Kubes *et al.*, 1993). These data indicate that cellular recruitment and, in particular, the crucial interaction of the leukocyte with endothelium, which are critical for the evolution of cell-mediated responses, can be modified by NO.

2.5 Effects of NO on T cell activation

NO exerts bi-phasic effects on T lymphocyte responsiveness. Initial observations described inhibition of *in vitro* antigen- or mitogen-driven T cell proliferation, either by NO donors or by macrophage-derived NO in co-cultures (Merryman *et al.*, 1993). Subsequently, it was established that low-dose NO significantly enhanced peripheral blood lymphocyte activation, measured by phytohaemagglutinin (PHA)-induced proliferation, increased glucose uptake, increased NF-κB binding activity and activation of protein tyrosine kinase p56[lck] (Lander *et al.*, 1993). Moreover, *in vitro* and *in vivo*, L-arginine enhances lymphocyte proliferation, and increases natural killer (NK) cell and lymphokine-activated killer activity (Park *et al.*, 1991). Recent studies in murine T cell clones have established that NO preferentially inhibits T_H1 clonal proliferation to antigen but had no effect on

T_H2 clones (Liew *et al.*, 1991; Taylor-Robinson *et al.* 1994; Wei *et al.*, 1995). Moreover, proliferative responses by spleen cells to mitogen and to staphylococcal superantigens are diminished in iNOS-deficient mice (Wei *et al.*, 1995; McInnes *et al.*, 1998). Thus, the local concentration of NO and the developmental phenotype influence the modulatory effect of NO on T cells. Cellular immune function may be further modified by NO through induction of apoptosis (Albina *et al.*, 1993).

2.6 Effects of NO on cytokine production

Cytokine production is influenced by NO, either directly or through modification of regulatory cell activity. T_H1 clones exhibit reduced IFN-γ production in the presence of NO, correlating with reduced proliferation (Taylor-Robinson *et al.*, 1994; Wei *et al.*, 1995). Whether NO induces reciprocal enhancement of T_H2 responses is unclear, although NO-donor-induced amplification of IL-4 secretion by T_H2 clones has recently been reported (Chang *et al.*, 1997). Similar observations have been made *in vivo*. iNOS-deficient mice generate exaggerated T_H1 responses, with increased IFN-γ generation during infection with *Staphylococcus aureus* (McInnes *et al.*, 1998) and *Leishmania major* (Wei *et al.*, 1995). Moreover, spleen cells from iNOS-deficient mice synthesize high levels of IFN-γ *a priori*, indicating that NO is normally required to regulate T_H1-type responses.

In addition to T cell cytokine regulation, NO is also implicated in monokine production. Increased TNFα production from peripheral blood mononuclear cells (PBMC) exposed to NO donors has been detected, although the cellular origin of TNFα in the PBMC was not specified (Lander *et al.*, 1993). Production of cytokine by purified blood monocyte/macrophages or macrophage cell lines has been variously reported to be suppressed or enhanced in the presence of exogenous NO (Deakin *et al.*, 1995; McInnes *et al.*, 1996). The mechanism underlying these observations is unknown but may reflect modification of transcription factors, such as NF-κB. We have recently demonstrated that NO induces TNFα synthesis by synovial tissues from rheumatoid arthritis (RA) patients, indicating that such observations probably have pathological relevance (McInnes *et al.*, 1996). Together these data indicate that complex feedback loops exist whereby the effector function of NO overlaps with its immunomodulatory role to 'fine-tune' ongoing immune responses.

2.7 NO and immune responses *in vivo*

Most evidence supports a critical role for NO during immune responses following infection. Early studies detected increased nitrate generation during septicaemia. NO has now been implicated in the response to a large number of organisms, including intracellular bacteria, fungi, protozoa, helminths and viruses. NO-dependent innate defence has been most studied in macrophages. In most cases, microbicidal activity is demonstrable *in vitro*, where it is inhibited by L-N^{ω}-

arginine analogues and is enhanced by addition of macrophage-activating factors, such as IFN-γ or LPS. Normally *in vivo*, T cells and macrophages cooperate to regulate NO synthesis through cytokine production. Thus, host responses to *L. major* are dependent on the generation of an effective T_H1 response, in which IL-12 and IFN-γ production leads to NO-mediated resistance. *L. major* infection in iNOS-deficient mice is of increased severity and mortality, despite the presence of an enhanced T_H1 response, indicating that NO is critical in host defence to this organism (Wei *et al.*, 1995). However, NO-mediated parasite killing can also proceed in the absence of T cells. *Listeria monocytogenes*-infected SCID mice, treated with aminoguanidine, exhibit increased mortality and enhanced recovery of viable listeria from spleens. IFN-γ production by NK cells is sufficient to confer resistance (Beckerman *et al.*, 1993). The leishmanicidal activity of NO derived from human macrophages has also been demonstrated (Kilbourn *et al.*, 1990).

NO may mediate host toxicity during infection. Elevated nitrate levels are detected in animals and humans with septicaemia. NOS inhibitors can reverse the hypotension of LPS-induced shock in rodents, although the effect is dose and time dependent (Vouldoukis *et al.*, 1995); preliminary trials in humans have indicated that some clinical features of septicaemia are NO dependent (Petros *et al.*, 1994). However, LPS-induced shock in iNOS knockout mice has yielded conflicting evidence, in favour of either a protective or a detrimental role for NO production (Wei, *et al.*, 1995; Gross, Kilbourn and Griffith, 1996), although differences in genetic strain between 'knockouts' may partially explain apparent discrepancies. The role of NO in Gram-positive infection is less clear. NO has been implicated in *S. aureus* killing by cytokineplasts from human neutrophils (Malawista, Montgomery and van Blaricom, 1996); and in a cell-free system, NO donors are bactericidal for *S. aureus*, although the time course of bacterial killing is delayed compared with that mediated by reactive oxygen intermediates (Kaplan *et al.*, 1996). *In vivo*, injection of certain staphylococcal exotoxins, such as TSST-1 or SEB, leads to a T lymphocyte-mediated shock syndrome in BALB/c mice, which can be exacerbated with exogenous NOS inhibitors (Florquin and Goldman, 1996). However, staphylococcal cell-wall components, such as peptidoglycan and lipoteichoic acid, synergistically induce multiple organ failure in rats by an NO-dependent mechanism (de Kimpe *et al.*, 1995). What is clear is that NO has 'double-edged' effects, and in some situations is aggressive to the host.

NO involvement in graft rejection is suggested by the nitrosylation of proteins during cardiac allograft rejection in rats (Lancaster *et al.*, 1992). iNOS expression is found at mRNA and protein levels in rejecting allografts, in both graft- and host-derived cells. Debate surrounds the net effect of NO production in rejection. Aminoguanidine treatment prolongs graft survival, reduces the histological grade of cellular infiltration and improves cardiac allograft contractility in rats (Worrall *et al.*, 1995). However, several studies have determined that iNOS inhibitors are deleterious to graft survival through removal of T cell regulatory activity attributable to NO. Moreover, BALB/c skin allograft rejection by iNOS-deficient mice is similar to that by heterozygote controls (Casey *et al.*, 1997). The precise role of NO production in alloreactivity is, therefore, unclear, although the latter data imply that NO production is not obligate in graft rejection.

The evidence reviewed above clearly implicated NO as an integral component of protective host immune responses. That NO is similarly involved in deleterious autoimmune responses, either as an aggressive or protective component, has been explored in several animal model systems. Murine disease resembling insulin-dependent diabetes mellitus (IDDM) occurs following inoculation with streptozocin, NO modified cytokine production within the pancreatic β islets and inhibition of NO production using NOS inhibitors led to delayed onset of disease, with attenuation of the pancreatic inflammatory infiltrate (Kolb and Kolb-Bachofen, 1992; Corbett *et al.*, 1993). Similarly, in the genetically predisposed non-obese diabetic (NOD) mouse model, transfer of NOD mouse spleen cells induced diabetes in irradiated recipients. The onset of disease was significantly delayed by amino-guanidine treatment (Okuda *et al.*, 1995). These findings implicate NO as an aggressor in IDDM pathogenesis. However, its role in experimental allergic encephalomyelitis (EAE) is more complex. NO production is up-regulated in EAE, and iNOS levels have been reported to correlate with disease severity (Zhao *et al.*, 1996). Whereas aminoguanidine was reported to inhibit clinical signs and progression of EAE in SJL mice and in Lewis rats (Ruuls *et al.*, 1996), paradoxical aggravation of EAE following administration of L^ω-arginine analogues has also been detected (Mulligan *et al.*, 1991). Suppression or aggravation of EAE by NOS inhibitors may depend on the mode of disease induction, or on the choice of inhibitor in T cell-induced, or myelin basic protein (MBP)-induced EAE. Such discrepancies again emphasize the double-edged effector function of NO as an immunosuppressor or a neurotoxin, dependent on subtle alterations of immunogen, inhibitor dosage and regimen.

NO has been implicated in immune complex-mediated disease. In pulmonary alveolitis induced by intratracheal injection of pre-formed immune complexes, NOS inhibitors reduced the severity of pulmonary haemorrhage and oedema formation. Similar inhibition of dermal vasculitis was observed. Moreover, a major component of this model is dependent on intact complement function, indicating that NO synthesis may interact with complement to mediate pathology (Mulligan *et al.*, 1991). Graft versus host disease (GVHD) in mice resembles the early stages of inflammatory bowel disease (IBD) or gut hypersensitivity syndromes such as coeliac disease. (CBA $\times$ BALB/c)F_1 recipients of CBA spleen cells develop GVHD, which is significantly retarded by L-NMMA treatment, with preservation of intestinal architecture and reduced density of intraepithelial lymphocyte infiltration (Garside *et al.*, 1992). However, it is unclear whether this effect operates primarily through immunoregulatory modification, or by haemodynamic effects in the mesenteric vasculature. NO production has been detected in human IBD, indicating that a role in human disease pathogenesis may exist (Broughton-Evans *et al.*, 1993). However, altered epithelial permeability found in IBD leads to increased exposure to bacteria and bacterial products within the lamina propria, with the potential for enhanced local NO production and consequent immunomodulation. Whether NO is ultimately protective or detrimental is, therefore, unclear.

Evidence for a role of NO in immune responses during inflammatory arthritis has been derived from several animal studies (Chapter 6). Adjuvant arthritis in rats bears histopathological similarities to RA. iNOS is detectable in synovial membrane and elevated levels of urinary and plasma nitrite are maximal after 14 days. Continuous administration of NOS inhibitors prevents or attenuates the clinical severity of arthritis, normalizes weight gain, reduces acute-phase response and retards erosive articular destruction (Ialenti, Moncada and DiRosa, 1993; Stefanovic-Racic *et al.*, 1994). Treatment during adjuvant priming alone is sufficient to confer subsequent reduction in disease severity, and anti-mycobacterial antigen-specific T cell responses are suppressed in treated rats. Similar data were obtained in streptococcal cell wall (SCW)-induced arthritis in rats, in which L-NMMA inhibited the onset and progression of arthritis (McCartney-Francis *et al.*, 1993). Administration of NOS inhibitors to MRL-MP-*lpr/lpr* mice suppressed the development of renal pathology and attenuated clinical and histological evidence of arthritis (Weinberg *et al.*, 1994). NO synthesis is closely linked to IL-12 production in this model, indicating that cytokine modulation by NO may complete a positive feedback loop, culminating in end-organ damage (Huang *et al.*, 1996). These data together implicate NO generation in articular pathology in rodents. We have recently demonstrated that NO is produced by macrophages and fibroblasts within the synovial membrane of patients with rheumatoid arthritis and have shown that such NO synthesis may enhance TNFα production, a cytokine which is critical to disease pathogenesis (see also Chapters 8 and 9 and McInnes *et al.*, (1996)).

The above observations clearly establish the production and regulatory importance of NO during immune responses in a variety of both antigen- and non-antigen-driven host responses *in vivo*.

2.8 Conclusions

NO represents a critical effector mechanism in a number of immune responses during infectious and autoimmune diseases. Complex feedback loops have evolved whereby NO may also regulate such responses. This tight balance of regulatory and effector function renders therapeutic intervention potentially difficult. Therefore, although iNOS inhibition appears attractive as an immunomodulatory target, careful estimation of its net effects in tissue pathology will be required. This will be particularly important in treatment of complex diseases such as the inflammatory arthropathies, in which multiple conflicting effects of NO in synovial membrane, cartilage and bone might be predicted.

Acknowledgements

The authors acknowledge financial support from the Wellcome Trust, the Nuffield Foundation and the Medical Research Council of Great Britain.

References

Albina, J. E., Cui, S., Mateo, R. B. and Reichner, J. S. (1993) Nitric oxide mediated apoptosis in murine peritoneal macrophages. *J. Immunol.* **150**, 5080–5085.

Amin, A. R., Di Cesare, P. E., Vyas, P. *et al.* (1995) The expression and regulation of nitric oxide synthase in human osteoarthritis affected chondrocytes: evidence for up-regulated neuronal NOS activity. *J. Exp. Med.* **182**, 2097–2102.

Assreuy, J., Cunha, F. Q., Liew, F. Y. and Moncada, S. (1993) Feedback inhibition of nitric oxide synthase activity by nitric oxide. *Br. J. Pharmacol.* **108**, 833–837.

Beckerman, K. P., Rogers, J. A., Corbett, R. D., Schreiber, M. L. and Unanue, E. R. (1993) Release of nitric oxide during the T cell independent pathway of macrophage activation. Its role in resistance to *Listeria monocytogenes. J. Immunol.* **150**, 888–895.

Bredt, D. S. and Snyder, S. H. (1994) Nitric oxide: a physiological messenger molecule. *Annu. Rev. Biochem.* **63**, 175–195.

Broughton-Evans, N. K., Evans, S. M., Hawkey, C. J. *et al.* (1993) Nitric oxide synthase activity in ulcerative colitis and Crohn's disease. *Lancet* **342**, 338–340.

Burkrinsky, M. I., Nottet, H. S. L. M., Schmidtmayerova, N. *et al.* (1995) Regulation of nitric oxide activity in HIV-infected monocytes: implications for HIV associated neurological disease. *J. Exp. Med.* **181**, 735–745.

Casey, J. J., Wei, X-Q., Orr, D. J. *et al.* (1997) Skin allograft rejection in mice lacking inducible nitric oxide synthase. *Transplantation*, in press.

Chang, R.-H., Lin Feng, M.-H., Liu, W.-H. and Lai, M.-Z. (1997) Nitric oxide increases interleukin-4 expression in T lymphocytes. *Immunology* **90**, 364–369.

Charles, I. G., Palmer, R. J., Hickery, M. S. *et al.* (1993) Cloning, characterisation and expression of a cDNA encoding an inducible nitric oxide synthase from human chondrocytes. *Proc. Natl. Acad. Sci., USA* **90**, 11419–11423.

Cho, H. J., Xie, Q. W., Calalcay, J., Mumford, R. A., Lee, T. D. and Nathan, C. (1992) Calmodulin is a subunit of nitric oxide synthase from macrophages. *J. Exp. Med.* **176**, 599–604.

Corbett, J. A., Mikhael, A., Shimizu, J. *et al.* (1993) Nitric oxide production in islets from nonobese diabetic mice, aminoguanidine-sensitive and -resistant stages in the immunological diabetic process. *Proc. Natl. Acad. Sci., USA* **90**, 8992–8995.

Deakin, A. M., Payne, A. N., Whittle, B. J. R. and Moncada, S. (1995) The modulation of IL-6 and TNFα release by nitric oxide following stimulation of J774 cells with LPS and IFN-γ. *Cytokine* **7**, 408–416.

de Kimpe, S. J., Kengatharan, M., Thiermann, C. and Vane, J. R. (1995) The cell wall components peptidoglycan and lipoteichoic acid from *Staphylococcus aureus* act in synergy to cause shock and multiple organ failure. *Proc. Natl. Acad. Sci., USA* **92**, 10359–10363.

Denis, M. (1991) Tumour necrosis factor and granulocyte colony stimulating factor stimulate human macrophages to restrict growth of virulent *Mycobacterium avium* and to kill avirulent *M. avium*: killing effector mechanism depends on generation of reactive nitrogen intermediates. *J. Leuk. Biol.* **49**, 380–387.

de Vera, M. E., Shapiro, R. A., Nussler, A. K. *et al.* (1996) Transcriptional regulation of human iNOS (NOS2) gene by cytokines. Initial analysis of the human NOS2 promoter. *Proc. Natl. Acad. Sci., USA* **93**, 1054–1059.

Di Rosa, M., Radomski, M., Carnuccio, R. and Moncada, S. (1990) Glucocorticoids inhibit the induction of nitric oxide synthesis in macrophages. *Biochem. Biophys. Res. Commun.* **172**, 1246–1252.

Dugas, B., Djavad Mossalayi, M., Damais, C. and Kolb, J. P. (1995) Nitric oxide production by human monocytes: evidence for a role of CD23. *Immunol. Today* **16**, 574–580.

Florquin, S. and Goldman, M. (1996) Immunoregulatory mechanisms of T cell dependent shock induced by a bacterial superantigen in mice. *Infect. Immun.* **64**, 3443–3445.

Garside, P., Hutton, A., Severn, A., Liew, F. Y. and Mowat, A. McI. (1992) Nitric oxide mediates intestinal pathology in graft versus host disease. *Eur. J. Immunol.* **22**, 2141–2145.

Geller, D. A., Nussler, A. K., Di Silvio, M. *et al.* (1993) Cytokines, endotoxin, and glucocorticoids regulate the expression of inducible nitric oxide synthase in hepatocytes. *Proc. Natl. Acad. Sci., USA* **90**, 522–526.

Gilbert, R. S. and Herschman, H. R. (1993) TGF beta differentially modulates the iNOS gene in distinct cell types. *Biochem. Biophys. Res. Commun.* **195**, 380–383.

Gross, S. S., Kilbourn, R. G. and Griffith, O. W. (1996) NO in septic shock: good, bad or ugly? Learning from iNOS knockouts. *Trend. Microbiol.* **4**, 47–49.

Huang, F.-P., Feng, G.-J., Lindop, G., Stott, D. and Liew, F. Y. (1996) The role of IL-12 and nitric oxide in the development of spontaneous autoimmune disease in MRL/MP- *lpr/lpr* mice. *J. Exp. Med.* **183**, 1447–1459.

Huang, P. L., Huang, Z., Mashimo, H. *et al.* (1995) Hypertension in mice lacking the gene for endothelial nitric oxide synthase. *Nature* **377**, 239–242.

Ialenti, A., Moncada, S. and Di Rosa, M. (1993) Modulation of adjuvant arthritis by endogenous nitric oxide. *Br. J. Pharmocol.* **110**, 701–706.

Ignarro, L. J., Buga, G. M., Wood, K. S., Byrns, R. E. and Chaudhuri, G. (1987) Endothelium derived relaxation factor produced and released from arteries and veins in nitric oxide. *Proc. Natl. Acad. Sci., USA* **84**, 9265–9269.

Isobe, K. and Nakashima, J. (1992) Feedback suppression of staphylococcal enterotoxin-stimulated T-lymphocyte proliferation by macrophages through inductive nitric oxide synthesis. *Infect. Immun.* **60**, 4832–4837.

Kamijo, R., Harada, H., Matsuyuma, T. *et al.* (1994) Requirement for transcription factor IRF-1 in NO synthase induction in macrophages. *Science* **263**, 1612–1615.

Kaplan, S. S., Lancaster, J. R., Basford, R. E. and Simmons, R. L. (1996) Effect of nitric oxide on staphylococcal killing and interactive effect with superoxide. *Infect. Immun.* **64**, 69–76.

Kilbourn, R. G., Jubran, A., Gross, S. S. *et al.* (1990) Reversal of endotoxin mediated shock by L-NMMA, an inhibitor of nitric oxide synthesis. *Biochem. Biophys. Res. Commun.* **172**, 1132–1138.

Kleinert, H., Euchenhofer, C., Ihrigbiedert, I. and Forstermann, U. (1996) Glucocorticoids inhibit the induction of iNOS by downregulating cytokine induced activity of transcription factor nuclear factor-κB. *Mol. Pharmacol.* **49**, 15–21.

Kolb, H. and Kolb-Bachofen, V. (1992) Nitric oxide: a pathogenetic factor in autoimmunity. *Immunol. Today* **13**, 157–160.

Kolyada, A. Y., Savikovsky, N. and Madias, N. E. (1996) Transcriptional regulation of the human iNOS gene in vascular smooth muscle cells and macrophages: evidence for tissue specificity. *Biochem. Biophys. Res. Commun.* **220**, 600–605.

Kubes, P., Kanwar, S., Niu, X. and Gaboury, J. P. (1993) Nitric oxide synthesis inhibition induces leukocyte adhesion via superoxide and mast cells. *FASEB J.* **7**, 1293–1299.

Kunz, D., Walker, G., Eberhardt, W. and Pfeilschifter, J. (1996) Molecular mechanisms of dexamethasone inhibition of nitric oxide synthase expression in IL-1 stimulated mesangial cells: evidence for the involvement of transcriptional and posttranscriptional regulation. *Proc. Natl. Acad. Sci., USA* **93**, 255–259.

Lancaster, J. R., Langrehr, J. M., Bergonia, H. A., Mutase, N., Simmons, R. L. and Hoffman, R. A. (1992) EPR detection of heme and non heme iron containing protein nitrosylation by nitric oxide during rejection of rat heart allograft. *J. Biol. Chem.* **267**, 10994–10998.

Lander, H. M., Sehajpal, P., Levine, D. M. and Novogrodsky, A. (1993) Activation of human peripheral blood cells by nitric oxide generating compounds. *J. Immunol.* **150**, 1509–1516.

Liew, F. Y. (1994) Regulation of nitric oxide synthesis in infectious and autoimmune diseases. *Immunol. Lett.* **43**, 95–98.

Liew, F. Y. and Cox, F. E. G. (1991) Non specific defence mechanism: the role of nitric oxide. *Immunol. Today* **12**, A17–A21.

Liew, F. Y., Li, Y., Severn, A., Millot, S., Schmidt, J., Salter, M. and Moncada, S. (1991) A possible novel pathway of regulation by murine T helper type-2 cells of a Th1 cell activity via the modulation of the induction of nitric oxide synthase in macrophages. *Eur. J. Immunol.* **21**. 2489–2494.

Lyons, C. R. (1995) The role of nitric oxide in inflammation. *Adv. Immunol.* **60**, 323–360.

MacMicking, J. D., Nathan, C., Hom, G. *et al.* (1995) Altered responses to bacterial infection and endotoxic shock in mice lacking inducible nitric oxide synthase. *Cell* **81**, 641–650.

Malawista, S. E., Montgomery, R. R. and van Blaricom, G. (1996) Evidence for nitrogen intermediates in killing of staphylococci in human neutrophil cytoplasts. *J. Clin. Invest.* **90**, 631–636.

McCartney-Francis, N., Allen, J. B., Mizel, D. E. *et al.* (1993) Suppression of arthritis by an inhibitor of nitric oxide synthase. *J. Exp. Med.* **178**, 749–754.

McInnes, I. B., Leung, B. P., Field, M. *et al.* (1996) Nitric oxide production in the synovial membranes of rheumatoid and osteoarthritis patients. *J. Exp. Med.* **184**, 1519–1524.

McInnes, I. B., Leung, B. P., Wei, X. Q., Gemmell, C. and Liew, F. Y. (1998) Staphylococcal arthritis in mice lacking inducible nitric oxide synthase. *J. Immunol.*, in press.

Mellilo, G., Musso, T., Taylor, L. S., Cox, G. W. and Varesio, L. (1995) A hypoxia responsive element mediates a novel pathway of activation of the inducible nitric oxide synthase promoter. *J. Exp. Med.* **182**, 1683–1693.

Merryman, P. F., Clancy, R. M., He, X. Y. and Abramson, S. B. (1993) Modulation of human T cell responses by nitric oxide and its derivative *S*-nitrosoglutathione. *Arthritis Rheum.* **36**, 1414–1422.

Mulligan, M. S., Heirel, J. M., Marletta, M. A. and Ward, P. A. (1991) Tissue injury caused by deposition of immune complexes is L-arginine dependent. *Proc. Natl. Acad. Sci., USA* **88**, 6338–6342.

Nathan, C. and Xie, Q.-W. (1994) Regulation of biosynthesis of nitric oxide. *J. Biol. Chem.* **269**, 13 725–13 728.

Okuda, Y., Nakatsuji, Y., Fujimura, H., Esumi, H., Ogura, T. and Yanagihara, T. (1995) Expression of the inducible isoform of nitric oxide synthase in the CNS of mice correlates with severity of actively induced EAE. *J. Neuroimmunol.* **62**, 103–112.

Palmer, R. M. J., Ferrige, A. G. and Moncada, S. (1987) Nitric oxide release accounts for the biologic activity of endothelium derived relaxing factor. *Nature* **327**, 524–526.

Park, K. G. M., Hayes, P. D., Garlick, P. J., Sewell, H. and Eremin, O. (1991) Stimulation of lymphocyte natural cytotoxicity by L-arginine. *Lancet* **337**, 645–646.

Petros, A., Lamdb, G., Leone, A., Moncada, S., Bennett, D. and Vallance, P. (1994) Effects of a nitric oxide synthase inhibitor in humans with septic shock. *Cardiovasc. Res.* **28**, 34–39.

Ruuls, S. R., van der Linden, S., Sontrop, K., Huitinga, I. and Dijkstra, C. D. (1996) Aggravation of experimental allergic encephalomyelitis (EAE) by administration of nitric oxide (NO) synthase inhibitors. *Clin. Exp. Immunol.* **103**, 467–474.

Schmidt, H. H. H. and Walter, U. (1994) NO at work. *Cell* **78**, 919–925.

Schneemann, M., Schoedon, G., Hoefer, S., Blau, N., Guerrero, L. and Schaffner, A. (1993) Nitric oxide synthase is not a constituent of the antimicrobial armature of human mononuclear phagocytes. *J. Inf. Dis.* **167**, 1358–1363.

Stefanovic-Racic, M., Meyers, K., Meschter, C., Coffey, J. W., Hoffman, R. A. and Evans, C. H. (1994) *N*-Monomethyl arginine, an inhibitor of nitric oxide synthase, suppresses the development of adjuvant arthritis in rats. *Arthritis Rheum.* **37**, 1062–1069.

Sunyer, T., Rothe, L., Jiang, X., Osdoby, P. and Collin-Osdoby, P. (1996) Proinflammatory agents, IL-8 and IL-10, upregulate inducible nitric oxide synthase expression and nitric oxide production in avian osteoclast like cells. *J. Cell. Biochem.* **60**, 469–483.

Tao, X. and Stout, R. (1993) T cell mediated cognate signalling of nitric oxide production by macrophages. Requirements for macrophage activation by plasma membranes isolated from T cells. *Eur. J. Immunol.* **23**, 2916–2921.

Taylor-Robinson, A. W., Liew, F. Y., Severn, A. *et al.* (1994) Regulation of the immune response by nitric oxide differentially produced by T helper type 1 and T helper type 2 cells. *Eur. J. Immunol.* **24**, 980–984.

Vouldoukis, I., Riveros-Moreno, V., Dugas, B. *et al.* (1995) The killing of *Leishmania major* by human macrophages is mediated by nitric oxide induced after ligation of the FcεRII/CD23 surface antigen. *Proc. Natl. Acad. Sci., USA* **92**, 7804–7808.

Wei, X. Q., Charles, I., Smith, A. *et al.* (1995) Altered immune responses in mice lacking inducible nitric oxide synthase. *Nature* **375**, 408–411.

Weinberg, J. B., Granger, D. L., Pisetsky, D. S. *et al.* (1994) The role of nitric oxide in the pathogenesis of spontaneous murine autoimmune disease expression in MRL-*lpr/lpr* mice, and reduction of spontaneous glomerulonephritis and arthritis by orally administered N^ω-monomethyl-L-arginine. *J. Exp. Med.* **179**, 651–660.

Worrall, N. K., Lazenby, W. D., Misko, T. P. *et al.* (1995) Modulation of *in vivo* alloreactivity by inhibition of inducible nitric oxide synthase. *J. Exp. Med.* **181**, 63–70.

Zembala, M., Siedlar, M., Marcinkiewicz, J. and Pryjma, J. (1994) Human macrophages are stimulated for nitric oxide release *in vitro* by some tumour cell lines but not by cytokines and lipopolysaccharide. *Eur. J. Immunol.* **24**, 435–439.

Zhao, W., Tilton, R. G., Corbett, J. A., McDaniel, M. L., Misko, T. P. and Williamson, J. R. (1996) Experimental allergic encephalomyelitis in the rat is inhibited by aminoguanidine, an inhibitor of nitric oxide synthase. *J. Neuroimmunol.* **64**, 123–133.

3

Bone biology and pathophysiological mechanisms of bone disease

R. GRAHAM G. RUSSELL, PETER CROUCHER,
BABATUNDE OYAJOBI, SHAMIM RAHMAN,
MICHAEL ROGERS and ANDREW SCUTT

3.1 Introduction

The physiological regulation of calcium homeostasis involves three main organs: the gut, the kidney and the skeleton. The fluxes of calcium and phosphate through these organs contributes to the integration of calcium metabolism throughout growth and adult life.

Until a few years ago the control of calcium metabolism and of skeletal remodelling was attributed mainly to the effects of systemic hormones, especially the calcium-regulating hormones, parathyroid hormone (PTH), 1,25-dihydroxy vitamin D (calcitriol) and calcitonin (CT). Other hormones, including thyroid and pituitary hormones and adrenal and gonadal steroids, also have major effects on the skeleton, as seen in clinical disorders in which their secretion is abnormally high or low. It is now realised that many additional factors, notably cytokines and growth factors, must also play a role in these processes, often by interacting locally with systemic hormones.

Bone is metabolically active throughout life. After skeletal growth is complete, remodelling of both cortical and trabecular bone continues and requires the coordinated actions of osteoclasts to remove bone and osteoblasts to replace it. Osteoclasts differentiate from haematopoietic stem cell precursors under the direction of factors that include cytokines such as colony-stimulating factors, interleukins and others. Osteoblasts within trabecular bone probably differentiate from stromal cell precursors in bone marrow and manufacture a complex extracellular matrix that subsequently mineralizes. Important factors for induction of new bone formation include members of the transforming growth factor beta (TGFβ) superfamily, which includes most of the bone morphogenetic proteins BMPs. Osteoblast activity is also influenced by insulin-like growth factors (IGFs), fibroblast growth factors (FGFs), PDGFs and prostaglandins. Parathyroid-related peptide (PTH-RP) and FGFs are also involved in cartilage differentiation; defects in their production or action are associated with chondrodysplasias. There are many ways in which these and other mediators contribute to the physiological regulation of bone metabolism and to the pathogenesis of skeletal diseases (Figure 3.1).

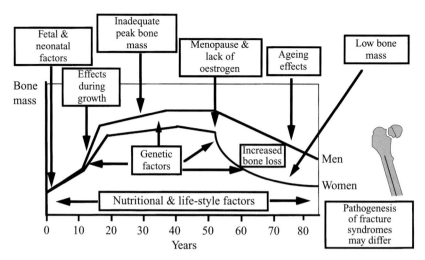

Figure 3.1. The pathogenesis of osteoporosis.

Monitoring of bone metabolism by biochemical means depends upon measurement of enzymes and proteins released during bone formation, (such as alkaline phosphatase, osteocalcin and collagen propeptides), and of degradation products produced during bone resorption. Tissue-specific processes can be measured by appropriate assays, such as pyridinoline crosslinks to reflect bone resorption.

3.2 Bone cell differentiation and function

3.2.1 Bone growth and remodelling

During growth, the skeleton enlarges in size. In long bones, this is achieved by the epiphysial growth plates producing increases in length, while increases in diameter result from deposition of new bone on the periosteal surfaces, accompanied by resorption from the endosteal surfaces.

During adult life, bone remodelling continues. In both cortical and trabecular bone, the process is initiated by the activation of osteoclasts, followed by the filling in of the resorption cavity by bone deposited by osteoblasts. The way in which these events are regulated is still only partially understood, but cytokines and growth factors are likely to be involved.

Intrinsic bone matrix proteins may themselves be regulators of cell function; for example, propeptides of collagen may act as endogenous regulators of procollagen synthesis within connective tissues. Osteocalcin, matrix Gla protein and the sialoproteins (e.g. osteopontin) may be chemoattractants for recruiting cells to the bone surface. Several matrix proteins, including collagen, osteonectin and osteopontin, have the cell receptor-binding domain characterized by the RGD amino acid sequence and can bind to integrins.

3.2.2 Bone resorption and osteoclasts

Osteoclasts are multinucleated cells derived from haematopoietic stem cells and are the major cells involved in bone resorption. Many cytokines can affect the differentiation and activity of osteoclasts and activate bone resorption (Figure 3.2). Prominent among these are proinflammatory cytokines such as IL-1 and IL-6: and TNFs.

3.2.3 Bone formation and osteoblasts

Osteoblasts in trabecular bone are derived from stromal stem cells, which reside in bone marrow (Figure 3.2). They are the major cells involved in bone formation, which results in deposition of matrix proteins and subsequent mineralization. Several growth factors can influence these events.

Important factors for induction of new bone formation include members of the TGFβ superfamily, which includes most of the BMPs. Other members of this family can induce cartilage formation, e.g. the cartilage-derived morphogenetic proteins (CDMPs), while PTH-RP and FGFs also influence cartilage differentiation; defects in their production are associated with chondrodysplasias. Osteoblast activity is also strongly influenced by IGFs I and II, FGFs and PDGFs. Osteoblasts themselves as well as marrow stromal cells are capable of producing a wide array of such factors, which can potentially act as autocrine and paracrine regulators of bone cell function. Several cytokines that can be produced by stromal cells and osteoblasts, such as CSFs and IL-6 and IL-11, may affect osteoclast recruitment rather than the function of mature cells. In some cases, systemic hormones such as PTH have been shown to be capable of influencing the production of these local factors (e.g. IL-6, prostaglandins, and IGFs from bone (Table 3.1 and Figure 3.3)).

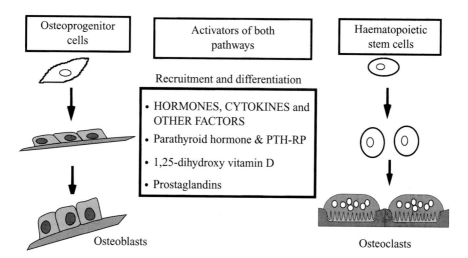

Figure 3.2. Factors that affect the differentiation of osteoclasts and osteoblasts.

Table 3.1. *Cytokines and growth factors that may affect bone and cartilage*

Group	Factors
Interleukins	1, 3, 4, 6, 8, 11, etc.
Interferons	α, γ
Growth factors	Fibroblast growth factors (FGFs acidic and basic)
	Insulin-like growth factors (IGF-I, IGF-II)
	Transforming growth factors (TGFα, TGFβ1–3)
	Bone morphogenetic proteins (BMPs 1–12+); cartilage-derived morphogenetic proteins (CDMPs 1–3)
	Epidermal growth factor (EGF)
	Platelet-derived growth factors (PDGF AA, BB, AB, etc.)
Colony-stimulating factors	Macrophage (M-CSF or CSF-1)
	Interleukin-3 (IL-3 or multi-CSF)
	Granulocyte-macrophage-CSF (GM-CSF)
	Stem cell factor
Neuropeptides	Substance P
	Vasoactive intestinal peptide (VIP)
	Calcitonin gene-related peptide (CGRP)
Others	Tumour necrosis factors (TNFα and TNFβ)
	Leukaemia inhibitory factors (LIFs)
	Parathyroid hormone-related protein (PTH-RP)
	Bradykinin
	Amylin
	Endothelin

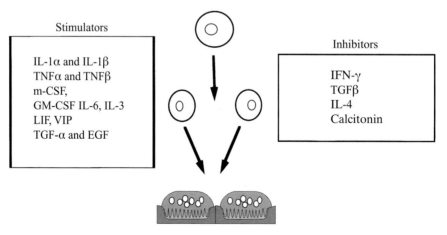

Figure 3.3. Factors that affect bone resorption. M-CSF, macrophage colony-stimulating factor; GM-CSF, granulocyte-macrophage colony-stimulating factor; VIP, vasoactive intestinal peptide.

3.2.4 Linking of bone resorption and bone formation

Many of the agents that cause bone resorption do not appear to act on osteoclasts directly but may produce their effects through osteoblasts or allied cells. There are numerous experimental demonstrations of potential interactions between osteoclasts and osteoblasts, but it is often questionable to what extent these reflect the mechanisms utilized *in vivo*. Co-culture experiments, for example, show that many agents that stimulate bone resorption do not appear to act directly on the mature osteoclast but require the presence of osteoblasts or related cells. These indirectly acting agents include PTH, 1,25-dihydroxy vitamin D, prostaglandins and bone-resorbing cytokines such as IL-1 and TNFs. However, the nature of this type of communication remains elusive; there is much current interest in the hypothesis that bone-resorbing agents generate an additional cellular messenger from osteo-blasts, which then acts on osteoclasts. The nature of these intercellular signals is not yet known, but communication of this type may be important in the maintenance of skeletal mass and in the phenomenon of coupling, which ensures that the processes of bone formation and bone destruction are more or less matched under many physiological and pathological conditions.

From published work, there is evidence for interactions of various types, for instance involving cell contact, and low-molecular-weight labile mediators such as NO, hydrogen peroxide and other reactive oxygen species. However, this raises the general problem of how short-lived, locally acting agents can account for the long-term coordination of the activity of osteoblasts and osteoclasts.

The role of cytokines derived from bone cells is potentially important but clearly defined roles remain to be established for many of them, and there may be new factors waiting to be discovered. Several known cytokines that can be produced by osteoblasts and stromal cells, such as colony-stimulating factors (CSFs), IL-6 and IL-11 may affect osteoclast recruitment rather than the function of mature cells.

It is also likely that growth factors within bone matrix, such as members of the TGFβ superfamily, which includes most of the BMPs, as well as the IGFs, FGFs, PDGFs and others may be involved in the regulation of cellular activity, but these processes are difficult to study by direct means. Such factors may be involved in the remodelling cycle within bone, during which the initial phase of osteoclastic resorption is followed by a more prolonged phase of bone formation mediated by osteoblasts. The extent of bone formation may be influenced by the exposure to matrix-derived growth factors. Regulation that is achieved by factors attached to matrix (e.g. FGF attached to heparin-like glycosaminoglycans) may be a mechanism for limiting cellular responses to specific sites within bone. This type of activity would then differ from that achieved by the release of soluble factors, which act within the local environment and beyond.

Another possibility is that the coordination is achieved not at the level of mature osteoclasts but at the level of differentiation of osteoclasts. For example, many of the bone-resorbing agents appear to stimulate the recruitment of osteoclasts from precursor cells (Figures 3.4 and 3.5).

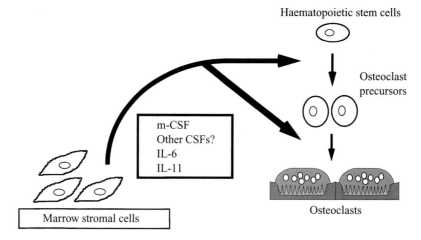

Figure 3.4. Interaction between stromal cells and osteoclast precursors.

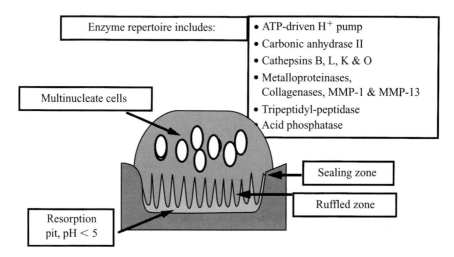

Figure 3.5. The main features of osteoclasts involved in bone resorption.

A further way in which the activity of osteoblasts and osteoclasts are coordinated may be through the generation of enzymes such as plasminogen activator (PA) from osteoblasts in response to bone-resorbing agents. Proteolysis of the surface matrix of bone may be an essential step in preparing it for subsequent resorption by incoming osteoclasts. Many of the agents that stimulate bone resorption (e.g. retinoids, PTH, 1,25-dihydroxy vitamin D, IL-1, etc.) can stimulate the production of plasminogen activator by osteoblast-like cells. Another mechanism may involve contraction of cells of the lining osteoblast layer in response to resorbing agents, such as PTH, thereby allowing access by osteoclasts.

Even though bone resorption induced by PTH or cytokines may involve the activation of osteoclasts by osteoblasts, there is a coupling of these cellular activities in the opposite direction in that after osteoclastic resorption is complete it is followed by deposition of new bone by osteoblasts. The amount of bone made under normal conditions corresponds very closely to the amount removed, so that in any remodelling cycle within bone the total amount of bone tends to remain constant. Even in conditions such as Paget's disease, where there seems to be a primary acquired abnormality of osteoclasts, the subsequent formative and reparative phase of bone deposition is still closely matched to the preceding resorption. The nature of these coupling mechanisms is still poorly understood, but they are very important since minor disturbances in them are likely to contribute to osteopenic or osteosclerotic states. Furthermore, any therapeutic attempts to increase bone mass (e.g. in osteoporosis) may be difficult to achieve unless these regulatory mechanisms can be circumvented.

3.3 Potential regulatory factors

Some of the regulatory factors that may have important effects on bone and cartilage are described below.

3.3.1 Interleukin 1

There are two major forms of IL-1, IL-1α and IL-1β, derived by complex proteolytic cleavage from larger precursors. IL-1 can be produced in large amounts by monocytes and macrophages and is a major mediator of inflammatory responses. Its many actions includes the induction of pyrogenic responses and the stimulation of an array of other cytokines, e.g. IL-2, IL-6 etc. IL-1 also stimulates the synthesis of prostaglandins, particularly via the inducible form of cyclooxygenase (Cox-2), which in turn is suppressible by glucocorticosteriods.

IL-1 can stimulate several types of cell (e.g. synovial cells, chondrocytes, fibroblasts) to secrete proteinases, including metalloproteinases (MMPs) such as collagenase (MMP-1) and stromelysin (MMP-3), as well as plasminogen activators. Collectively these enzymes can contribute to the breakdown of connective tissue matrices. IL-1 is one of the most potent known inducers of bone resorption and was one of the first osteoclast-activating factors (OAFs) to be characterized. IL-1 causes hypercalcaemia when injected and may account for bone resorption associated with monocytic leukaemias and inflammatory erosive conditions in bone, e.g. osteomyelitis, RA and periodontal disease. IL-1 also has complex effects, often inhibitory, on the production of matrix components, including collagen, osteocalcin and proteoglycans.

3.3.2 Interleukin 1 receptor antagonist

A third member of the IL-1 gene family located in the same gene cluster on chromosome 2 is the IL-1 receptor antagonist (IL-1 ra), which acts as a naturally occurring inhibitor of IL-1 by blocking binding of IL-1 to its receptor. IL-1 ra can inhibit the bone loss occurring after ovariectomy in rats, suggesting that IL-1 mediates the bone loss seen after oestrogen deprivation. IL-1 ra has also been studied as a therapeutic agent in humans against septic shock and in RA.

3.3.3 *Tumour necrosis factors*

TNF exists in two forms, TNFα and TNFβ, which display extensive homology and have a very similar spectrum of activity to each other and to IL-1.

TNFα was originally isolated on the basis of activity termed cachectin and was thought to be responsible for weight loss in tumour-bearing animals. TNFβ, also known as lymphotoxin, is derived from T lymphocytes and may mediate their cytotoxicity.

The effects of TNFs on connective tissues are very similar to those of IL-1 and include induction of prostaglandin and MMP synthesis, the stimulation of bone and cartilage resorption, and mitogenesis. On a molar basis, IL-1 is more potent than TNFα, but the two can act in a synergistic fashion under certain circumstances. They can also induce the production of each other and of other cytokines.

The TNF molecules exist as trimers and their biological activities can be neutralized by soluble shed receptors, of which there are two forms (p55 or p75). Therapeutic neutralization of TNF activity can be achieved with antibodies or with soluble receptor constructs and has shown encouraging clinical responses in patients with RA.

3.3.4 *Interleukin 6*

IL-6 can be produced by many types of connective tissue cell, including human bone and cartilage cells, and by monocytes. IL-6 is now known to be responsible for several biological activities previously ascribed to separate factors and has some important overlapping activities with IL-1 and TNF. IL-1, TNF and LPS (endotoxin) are strong inducers of the production of IL-6 from several cell types, including bone cells, so that some biological effects attributable to IL-1 and TNF may be mediated via IL-6. The most important of these may be the augmentation of hepatic acute-phase protein synthesis; IL-6 is probably an important mediator of the acute-phase response.

The function of the large amount of IL-6 that can be produced in bone is not yet clarified. In mice, IL-6 can cause hypercalcaemia and may stimulate bone resorption, but its role in humans is less clear. It appears to be an important growth factor for myeloma cells, and antibodies to IL-6 can produce a therapeutic response in myeloma patients. Mice with the IL-6 gene ablated show less bone loss after ovariectomy, suggested that oestrogens may also act via IL-6.

3.3.5 *Colony-stimulating factors*

CSFs play a key role in haemopoietic differentiation, as does IL-1, and may be induced by other cytokines, e.g. TNF and IL-1 (Figure 3.6). Granulocyte-macro-

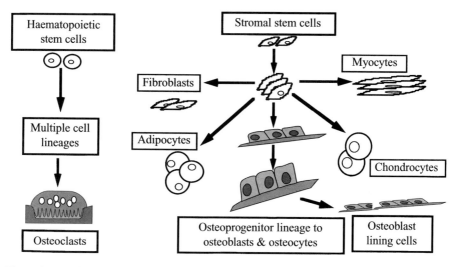

Figure 3.6. Differentiation to osteoclasts and osteoblasts.

phage CSF (GM-CSF) and macrophage CSF (M-CSF) can also stimulate bone resorption *in vitro*; this may be attributable to their effects on osteoclast generation, since both can be shown to stimulate the generation of osteoclast-like cells from bone marrow cultures. Both can also be produced by osteoblast-like cells, which raises the interesting possibility that bone cells can influence haematopoiesis in the bone micro-environment. Lack of biologically active M-CSF resulting from a gene defect is responsible for defective macrophage and osteoclast differentiation in the *op/op* mouse, which has an osteopetrotic phenotype. The bone lesions can be reversed by administration of M-CSF.

3.3.6 Interferon gamma

Interferons were originally defined by their ability to inhibit viral replication but are known to have many other effects, particularly on cellular proliferation and differentiation, which has led to their therapeutic use as anti-tumour agents and as immunomodulators.

IFN-γ, while sharing some properties with other interferons, appears to differ from IFN-α and IFN-β in terms of its effects on connective tissues. For example, IFN-γ inhibits bone resorption induced by IL-1 or TNF, whereas it has less effect on resorption stimulated by the classical calciotrophic hormones or 1,25 dihydroxy vitamin D.

IFN-γ also opposes other actions of IL-1 and TNF, for example on cell proliferation, on cartilage resorption and on metalloproteinase production by chondrocytes. In these respects, it can be viewed as a potential natural antagonist to IL-1 and TNF. IL-4 may have similar effects.

INF-γ also induces the expression of MHC class 2 (HLA-DR) antigens on connective tissue cells, including synovial cells, bone cells and chondrocytes, as it does on macrophages. These changes may allow these connective tissue cells to present antigens and to participate in immune responses, or in other forms of intercellular communication.

3.3.7 Fibroblast growth factors

FGFs are members of a large family of related peptides (15–16 kDa) that are mitogenic for many cell types, including fibroblasts and osteoblasts.

There are acidic and basic forms of FGF, based on isoelectric points, and they share some homology with IL-1. Acidic FGF is derived mainly from neural tissue, but basic FGF is one of the heparin-binding growth factors; it appears to be produced by many cell types and is present in bone matrix.

FGFs are powerful angiogenic factors and are important during embryological development (e.g. during limb bud development), during endochondral ossification and in various pathological states (Figures 3.7 and 3.8).

The importance of FGF in the development of the growth plate has been dramatically illustrated by the identification of the genetic defect underlying achondroplasia as a point mutation causing an amino acid substitution in the transmembrane domain of the type 3 form of the FGF receptor. Achondroplasia is a common form of dominantly inherited dwarfism that occurs by new mutations and it is, therefore, remarkable that the genotype seems to be the same in all patients studied.

3.3.8 Insulin-like growth factors (IGFs) and their binding factors

IGFs, as the name implies, are growth factors that share some structural and biological properties with insulin; they were originally isolated from serum. IGF-I formerly known as somatomedin C, stimulates the replication of bone cells and chondrocytes and increases production of matrix constituents. Both IGF-I and IGF-II are produced within bone itself, and their activity is modulated by specific binding proteins, of which there are at least six, some of which are also under endocrine control. There may be important species differences in the regulation by IGFs, with IGF-II dominating in human bone, while IGF-I is the major endogenous IGF in rat bone (Figures 3.7 and 3.8).

3.3.9 Transforming growth factor β

The TGFβ family are members of a much larger gene family and are produced by a variety of cells and tissues that include bone. The TGFβ family comprises homodimeric polypeptides (25 kDa) that exist in at least three isoforms (TGFβ 1, 2 and 3) with different primary sequences but similar biological activities. TGFβ members are thought to be important in embryological development and differentia-

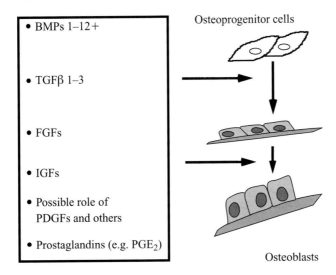

Figure 3.7. Factors that affect differentiation to and activity of osteoblasts.

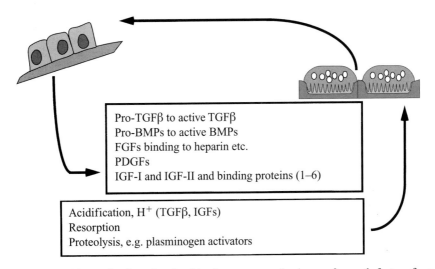

Figure 3.8. Possible mechanisms involved in the storage and release of growth factors from bone matrix.

tion as well as in connective tissue repair and fibrosis. They are one of the most important family of regulatory cytokines in connective tissues and bone.

In vitro TGFβ stimulates the synthesis of extracellular matrix components such as type I collagen and fibronectin. In the presence of EGF, TGFβ stimulates the proliferation of a variety of connective tissue cell types including bone cells. When injected *in vivo*, TGFβ induces a wound repair response that includes fibrosis and angiogenesis. TGFβ may be involved in inducing pathological fibrosis, for example in liver cirrhosis. When TGFβ is injected in or around existing bone it produces a remarkable induction of new bone (Figures 3.7 and 3.8).

TGFβ is one of the few agents known to inhibit the production from fibroblasts of proteinases such as plasminogen activator and stromelysin (MMP-3), which may be involved in the degradation of extracellular matrix proteins. TGFβ also stimulates the production of inhibitors of plasminogen activators (known as PAIs) and of metalloproteinases (tissue inhibitors of metalloproteinases, TIMPs). These actions of TGFβ may be important in the maintenance of the integrity of extracellular matrix and, in concert with its effects on matrix synthesis, may promote tissue repair.

TGFβ is produced in latent form and can be activated by exposure to an acid environment. The latency arises through the existence of pro-forms, through binding to α_2-macroglobulin, and through association with a large protein (135 kDa) denoted LAP (latency associated protein). It has been suggested, therefore, that active TGFβ may be released from bone matrix during resorption and thus be available to affect both osteoblastic and osteoclastic activity.

The TGFβ class of growth factor also includes the bone-inductive factors known as BMPs.

3.3.10 Bone morphogenetic proteins and cartilage-derived morphogenetic proteins

BMPs derive their given names as factors present in demineralized bone matrix that can induce the formation of new cartilage and bone when implanted into various non-skeletal sites *in vivo*. The characterization of BMPs was a difficult task, partly because of the limitations imposed by the laborious bioassay. BMPs are now known to be important in regulating the differentiation of skeletal and other tissues and may eventually be of therapeutic use, for example to promote repair of fractures and skeletal defects.

Apart from BMP-I, which curiously turns out to be a proteinase capable of cleaving the C-terminal propeptide from type 1 collagen, the remaining dozen or so BMPs described are members of the TGFβ family. This family also includes the recently identified CDMPs, of which three have been described. These are involved in the differentiation of cartilage. Abnormalities in CDMP-1 are associated with brachypodism in mice.

3.3.11 Parathyroid hormone-related peptides

The discovery of PTH-RP has provided a rational basis for understanding the pathophysiology of hypercalcaemia of malignancy, for which it has been recognized for a long time that factors resembling PTH itself might be involved.

PTH-RP peptides are produced by non-parathyroid tissues such as breast and skin; there may also be a fetal form of PTH. In hypercalcaemia associated with malignant disease, PTH-RP has been implicated particularly in breast tumours and squamous cell carcinomas.

Several closely related PTH-RP peptides have now been identified as single chain peptides containing about 140 amino acid residues. The N-terminal portion shows considerable homology with PTH itself; at present only a single receptor for PTH and PTH-RP has been identified.

An unexpected finding has been that mice with deletion of either the PTH-RP gene or the PTH–PTH-RP receptor gene show defects in the growth plate. Moreover, a rare inherited form of dwarfism in humans, Jansen type metaphysial dysplasia, is associated with a substitution of histidine by arginine at a critical position (223) in the PTH–PTH-RP receptor.

These observations, together with the evidence that PTH-RPs are produced by bone and cartilage cells, indicate that PTH-RP may be an important autocrine and paracrine regulator within bone and cartilage.

3.3.12 *Prostaglandins and eicosanoids*

It has been known for a very long time that prostaglandins have effects on bone under experimental conditions, but their physiological and pathological significance is still not fully resolved. There have been two major recent developments in this field that are likely to have a significant impact on future research. The first is the discovery of a second form of cyclooxygenase (COX-2), inducible by cytokines and inhibitable by glucocorticoids. Non-steroidal anti-inflammatory drugs (NSAIDs) can now be reclassified based on their different inhibitory potencies on COX-1 and COX-2. The second is the characterization of the prostanoid receptors, of which at least four major subtypes exist.

Prostaglandin E_2 is one of the most potent of the prostanoids for induction of bone resorption. The ability of several agents to stimulate bone resorption (e.g. TGFβ, complement components, thrombin, IL-1, TNF) may be mediated, in part at least, by increased prostaglandin synthesis, in many cases probably by inducing synthesis of COX-2. In turn, production of several of these cytokines may be influenced by prostaglandins. In contrast, low concentrations of some prostanoids may inhibit osteoclast actions by directly altering cell mobility.

Prostaglandins, such as prostacyclin (PGI$_2$), may be involved in the response of bone to mechanical stress and may help to mediate the bone loss associated with immobilization. They may be involved in the localized bone resorption associated with periodontal disease, neoplasia and inflammation. The chronic administration of prostaglandins *in vivo* may lead to enhanced periosteal and endosteal apposition of bone, for example in children with patent ductus arteriosus and in experimental animals. These potential anabolic effects of prostaglandins have not yet been exploited clinically.

Products of the lipoxygenase pathways, such as leukotrienes, also appear to have marked effects on bone cell function and may activate osteoclasts directly. Some of these products may be generated in response to proinflammatory cytokines and other agents.

3.4 Factors affecting the action of cytokines and growth factors

3.4.1 Cytokine and growth factor receptors

Following the identification of the many cytokines and growth factors, their receptors have now been extensively characterized. These too fall into several classes and in many cases there is more than one receptor isoform for each agonist.

The cellular distribution of receptors helps to determine tissue responsiveness to these factors, and receptor expression itself is modulated by exposure to hormones and cytokines.

In many cases, receptors can be shed by proteolytic action from cell surfaces, and shed receptors may have important roles in neutralizing the activity of extracellular cytokines.

3.4.2 Role of cytokine gene polymorphisms

There is increasing evidence for cytokine gene polymorphisms, which may be linked to occurrence or severity of inflammatory or infectious disease. There are examples of such polymorphisms in the genes encoding IL-1α and IL-1β, IL-1 ra and TNFα. These genetic variants may result in differences in cytokine production.

3.5 Some specific aspects of the regulation of bone and cartilage metabolism in health and disease

3.5.1 Mechanical effects on bone

Mechanical forces exert strong influences on bone shapes and modelling. Early responses to mechanical loading may include early induction of prostacyclin synthesis and NO production, and later increases in IGFs and changes in amino acid transporters; eventually increases in new bone formation occur.

3.5.2 Other cellular interactions in bone

There are many potential interactions between the haematopoietic, stromal and immune systems and bone that may be important within the microenvironment of bone in terms of osteoclast recruitment, bone resorption, osteoblastic activity and haematopoiesis. Many different mediators and mechanisms are likely to be involved in the interactions between these accessory cells and bone and these may, therefore, play a role in the physiology and pathology of bone. In cancer, there may be bidirectional interactions between tumour cells and bone.

3.5.3 Systemic or local effects of cytokines

Several of the cytokines may have systemic effects as well as local effects at their site of production. Appropriate immunoassays and bioassays demonstrate that cytokines such as IL-1, TNF, IGF-I, IFNs and IL-6 are present in the systemic circulation, particularly in disease states (e.g. infections, burns, shock, hepatic failure, etc.). In spite of this, not all potential target tissues display a response. For example, changes in bone and cartilage are not seen in all these clinical situations.

The responsiveness of each tissue is likely to depend upon many variables, including the concentration of individual cytokines present, the relative amount of different cytokines, the potential synergisms and antagonisms among them, the degree of receptor modulation (e.g. by glucocorticoids), and the presence of specific inhibitors (such as shed receptors), and autoantibodies.

3.5.4 Lessons from transgenic animals

Since there are so many factors that can potentially act on bone, a major task in contemporary research is to determine how these agents interact and which are the most important under physiological conditions and in different disease states. This task is only just beginning. As already illustrated by M-CSF and PTH-RP, gene knockouts or genetic defects can be very informative.

Some of the transgenic models do not show the expected phenotype, for example the lack of a skeletal phenotype in a TGFβ knockout and the occurence of osteopenia associated with overexpression of the IL-4 gene in mice.

3.5.5 Interactions between oestrogens and cytokines, and their relevance to osteoporosis

Osteoporosis is clearly a multifactorial disorder and much remains to be learnt about the many pathogenic processes that eventually contribute to the bone loss that leads to osteopenia. Although the majority of patients with osteoporosis do not display florid disturbances in immune function, abnormalities in immunoregulation, arising from oestrogen deficiency, may contribute to bone loss in osteoporosis.

The effects of oestrogen in bone are of particular interest in relation to the loss of bone after the menopause in women and the therapeutic use of oestrogen to prevent this. Earlier explanations for the bone-sparing effect of oestrogen include a stimulation of calcitonin production and a resulting decrease in bone resorption or, alternatively, enhanced availability of 1,25-dihydroxy vitamin D$_3$ leading to increased intestinal calcium absorption. More important effects may include actions on the immune system, culminating, for example, in an inhibition of the release of promoters of bone resorption, as well as direct effects on bone cells through recently discovered oestrogen receptors. Despite earlier negative reports, there is now evidence that oestrogen receptors exist in bone, although in low concentrations. In osteoporosis, changes in IL-1 production have been claimed to occur. The production of several cytokines (IL-1, TNF, GM-CSF) from monocytes is increased after the menopause and can be suppressed by administration of oestrogens. Our own studies show that the production of TNF from peripheral blood mononuclear cells can be markedly inhibited by oestrogens in post-menopausal women, but not in pre-menopausal women or men.

There is now, therefore, considerable experimental as well as clinical evidence to suggest that at least some of the effects of oestrogen on bone (and other tissues) may be mediated by oestrogen-dependent changes in the production of cytokines and other mediators. The production of cytokines such as IL-1, TNFα, IL-6 and GM-CSF, which can all potentially enhance production of osteoclasts and bone resorption, can be suppressed in monocytes by physiological doses of oestrogen. In mice, ovariectomy does not lead to normal rates of bone loss in mice with an IL-6 gene knockout, while in rats, administration of a IL-1 receptor antagonist reduces bone loss after ovariectomy.

It is also possible that oestrogens have significant anabolic effects on bone. Oestrogens can affect the proliferation of osteoprogenitor cells and osteoblast-like cells. Part of this effect may be mediated by oestrogen altering the production by osteoblasts of a number of potentially locally acting growth factors such as IGFs and their binding proteins, and of TGFβ by bone cells. Oestrogens may also influence the production of prostaglandin E_2.

The pathogenesis of osteoporosis in men is less well studied than in women but is clinically important, with secondary causes, for example hypogonadism, being common. The effects of androgens on cytokines are less well characterized.

3.6 Prospects for the future

The rapidly accumulating new knowledge about the possible multiple regulatory mechanisms within bone should aid the understanding of physiological bone remodelling and also offer potential explanations for the changes in bone turnover

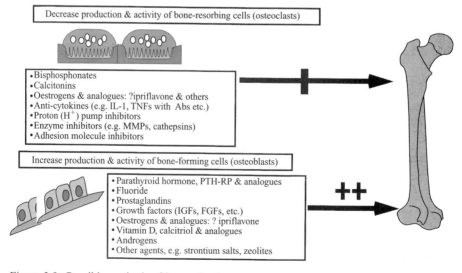

Figure 3.9. Possible methods of increasing bone mass.

seen in a variety of disease states. This knowledge will be important in devising new therapeutic strategies to control bone formation and resorption based on these novel regulatory mechanisms (Figure 3.9).

Further reading

Blakemore, A. I. F., Tarlow, J. K., Cork, M. J., Gordon, C., Emery, P. and Duff, G. (1994) Interleukin-1 receptor antagonist gene polymorphism as a severity factor in systemic lupus erythematosus. *Arthritis Rheum.* **37**, 1380–1385.

Border, W. A. and Noble, N. A. (1994) Transforming growth factor beta in tissue fibrosis. *N. Eng. J. Med.* **331**, 1286–1292.

Callard, R. and Gearing, A. (1994) *The Cytokine Facts Book*. Academic Press, London.

Eriksen, E. F., Colvard, D. S., Berg, N. J. *et al.* (1988) Evidence of estrogen receptors in normal human osteoblast-like cells. *Science* **241**, 84–86.

Felix, R., Cecchini, M. G. and Fleisch, H. (1990) Macrophage colony stimulating factor restores *in vivo* bone resorption in the *op/op* osteopetrotic mouse. *Endocrinology* **127**, 2592–2594.

Girasole, G., Jilka, R. L., Passeri, G. *et al.* (1992) 17beta-Estradiol inhibits interleukin-6 production by bone marrow-derived stromal cells and osteoblasts *in vitro*: a potential mechanism for the antiosteoporotic effect of estrogens. *J. Clin. Invest.* **89**, 883–891.

Girasole, G., Passeri, G., Jilka, R. L. and Manolagas, S. C. (1994) Interleukin-11 a new cytokine critical for osteoclast development. *J. Clin. Invest.* **93**, 1516–1524.

Gowen, M., Wood, D. D., Ihrie, E. J., McGuire, M. K. B. and Russell, R. G. G. (1983) An interleukin-1-like factor stimulates bone resorption *in vitro*. *Nature* **306**, 378–380.

Gowen, M., Nedwin, G. E. and Mundy, G. R. (1986) Preferential inhibition of cytokine-stimulated bone resorption by recombinant interferon gamma. *J. Bone Min. Res.* **1**, 469–473.

Ho, K. K. Y. and Weissberger, A. J. (1992) Impact of short-term estrogen administration of growth hormone secretion and action – distinct route-dependent effects on connective and bone tissue metabolism. *J. Bone Min. Res.* **7**, 821–827.

Jilka, R. L., Hangoc, G., Girasole, G. *et al.* (1992) Increased osteoclast development after estrogen loss – mediation by interleukin-6. *Science* **257**, 88–91.

Klein, B., Wijdenes, J., Zhang, X.-G. *et al.* (1991) Murine anti-interleukin-6 monoclonal antibody therapy for a patient with plasma cell leukemia. *Blood* **78**, 1198–1204.

Lynch, S. E., Williams, R. C. and Polson, A. M. (1989) A combination of platelet-derived and insulin-like growth factors enhances priodontal regeneration. *J. Clin. Periodontol.* **16**, 545–548.

Manolagas, S. C. and Jilka, R. L. (1995) Emerging insights into the pathophysiology of osteoporosis. *N. Engl. J. Med.* **332**, 305–311.

Morrison, N. A., Qi, J. C., Tokita, A. *et al.* (1994) Prediction of bone density from vitamin-D receptor alleles. *Nature* **367**, 284–287.

Mundy, G. R. (1995) *Bone Remodeling and its Disorders*. Martin Dunitz.

Pacifici, R. (1992) Is there a causal role for IL-1 in postmenopausal bone loss. *Calcif. Tiss. Int.* **50**, 295–299.

Pacifici, R., Rifas, L., Teitelbaum, S. *et al.* (1987) Spontaneous release of interleukin 1 from human blood monocytes reflects bone formation in idiopathic osteoporosis. *Proc. Natl. Acad. Sci., USA* **84**, 4616–4620.

Pacifici, R., Rifas, L., McCracken, R. *et al.* (1989) Ovarian steroid treatment blocks a postmenopausal increase in blood monocyte interleukin 1 release. *Proc. Natl. Acad. Sci. USA* **86**, 2398–2402.

Pacifici, R., Vannice, J. L., Rifas, L. and Kimble, R. B. (1993) Monocytic secretion of interleukin-1 receptor antagonist in normal and osteoporotic women: effects of menopause and estrogen/progesterone therapy. *J. Clin. Endocrinol. Metab.* **77**, 1135.

Passeri, G., Girasole, G., Jilka, R. L. and Manolagas, S. C. (1993) Increased interleukin-6 production by murine bone marrow and bone cells after estrogen withdrawal. *Endocrinology*, **133**, 822–828.

Pioli, G., Basini, G., Pedrazzoni, M. *et al.* (1992) Spontaneous release of interleukin-1 and interleukin-6 by peripheral blood mononuclear cells after oophorectomy. *Clin. Sci.*, **83**, 503–507.

Poli, V., Balena, R., Fattori, E. *et al.* (1994) Interleukin-6 deficient mice protected from bone loss caused by estrogen depletion *EMBO J.* **13**, 1189–1196.

Raisz, L. G. (1988) Local and systemic factors in the pathogenesis of osteoporosis. *N. Engl. J. Med.* **318**, 818–828.

Ralston, S. H., Russell, R. G. G. and Gowen, M. (1990) Estrogen inhibits release of tumor necrosis factor from peripheral blood mononuclear cells in postmenopausal women. *J. Bone Min. Res.* **5**, 983–988.

Rickard, D. J., Russell, R. G. G. and Gowen, M. (1992) Oestradiol inhibits the release of tumor necrosis factor but not IL-6 from adult human osteoblasts *in vitro*. *Osteoporosis Int.* **2**, 94–102.

Rousseau, F., Bonaventure, J., Legeai-Mallet, L. *et al.* (1994) Mutations in the gene encoding fibroblast growth factor receptor-3 in achondroplasia. *Nature* **371**, 252–254.

Russell, R. G. G. (1990) Bone cell biology: the role of cytokines and other mediators. *Osteoporosis 1990.* (ed. R. Smith), pp. 9–33. Royal College of Physicians, London.

Schipani, E., Kruse, K. and Juppner, H. A. (1995) A constitutively active mutant PTH-PTHrP receptor in Jansen type metaphyseal chondrodysplasia. *Science* **268**, 98–100.

Skodjt, H. and Russell, R. G. G. (1992) Bone cell biology and the regulation of bone turnover. In *Cytokine and Bone Metabolism*. (ed. M. Gowen), pp. 1–170. CRC Press, Baton Rouge, FL.

Stahl, N. and Yancopoulos, G. D. (1993) The alphas, betas, and kinases of cytokine receptor complexes. *Cell* **74**, 587–590.

Stock, J. L., Coderse, J. A., McDonald, B. and Rosenwasser, L. J. (1989) Effects of estrogen *in vivo* and *in vitro* on spontaneous interleukin-1 release by monocytes from postmenopausal women. *J. Clin. Endocrinol. Metab.* **68**, 364–368.

Tarlow, J. K., Blakemore, A. I. F., Lennard, A. *et al.* (1993) Polymorphism in human IL-1 receptor antagonist gene intron 2 is caused by variable numbers of an 86-bp tandem repeat. *Hum. Genet.* **91**, 403–404.

Turner, R. T., Riggs, B. L. and Spelsberg, T. C. (1994) Skeletal effects of estrogen. *Endocrine Rev.* **15**, 275–300.

SECTION II

Nitric oxide in arthritis

4

Nitric oxide and blood flow in arthritis

JOHN C. LOCKHART, LORRAINE MCMURDO and
WILLIAM R. FERRELL

4.1 Introduction

The importance of NO in modulating vascular reactivity has long been recognized. Initially referred to as endothelial-derived relaxing factor (EDRF), it is now widely accepted that NO fulfils this vasodilating role in most vascular beds (Ignarro *et al.*, 1987), including that of synovial joints (Najafipour and Ferrell, 1993). It is synthesized in the endothelial cells lining the blood vessels and is released to diffuse into adjacent vascular smooth muscle cells where it stimulates cGMP production via activation of guanylyl cyclase. The resulting increase in intracellular levels of cGMP acts to relax the vascular smooth muscle and thereby induce vasodilatation (Chapters 1 and 2).

Rheumatoid arthritis (RA) is a chronic inflammatory disease of uncertain aetiology that manifests itself by joint pain and swelling, synovial hyperaemia and cartilage destruction. Macrophages, neutrophils and lymphocytes migrate into the the inflamed synovium, where there is evidence that cytokines are released (Arend and Dayer, 1990). Stadler *et al.* (1991) first implicated NO in joint inflammation by demonstrating that the cytokine IL-1 induced NO formation in cultures of rabbit articular chondrocytes, as did lipopolysaccharide. This is supported by more recent *in vivo* work (Ialenti, Moncada and DiRosa, 1993; McCartney-Francis *et al.*, 1993; Stefanovic-Racic *et al.*, 1994) in which non-specific inhibitors of NO synthesis substantially supressed development of joint inflammation in chronic models of arthritis. The elevated levels of NO reported in both the serum and synovial fluid of patients with RA compared with controls (Farrell *et al.*, 1992; Ueki *et al.*, 1996) is consistent with a proinflammatory role for NO in joint disease. The fact the NO levels were also greater in synovial fluid than in matched serum samples suggests that NO is generated locally within the joint during inflammation, and that spillover of this contributes to the elevated serum NO levels in RA. Moreover, the increased serum levels of inflammatory cytokines found in these patients particularly implicates iNOS as being at least partly responsible for the generation of the raised NO levels during joint inflammation. By specifically targeting iNOS using selective inhibitors in rats, Connor *et al.* (1995) demonstrated that joint inflammation could be attenuated in adjuvant-

induced arthritis, thus further supporting a critical role for iNOS in the inflammatory processes.

4.2 Sites of NO release in the joint

Given the relatively short half life of NO (<1 min), local generation of NO within
the joint is necessary for its participation in intra-articular physiological and patho-
physiological processes. Potential sources of NO in diathrodial joints include not
only the endothelial cells of the synovial vasculature but also chondrocytes, synoviocytes and, possibly, ligament cells. The nerves innervating the joint could also be a
source of NO, since nNOS is widely distributed in the peripheral nervous system
(Bredt, Hwang and Snyder, 1990) and is released from non-adrenergic non-choliner-
gic fibres (reviewed by Grozdanovic, Bruning and Baumgarten, 1994). Indeed, the
greater proportion of cNOS activity in humans has been ascribed to nNOS (Knowles
and Moncada, 1994). A neural source of NO has also been implicated from functional
studies previously undertaken in our laboratory (see below).

Cultures of articular chondrocytes and synovial fibroblasts from rabbits have
been shown to synthesize large amounts of NO when stimulated with proinflammatory cytokines (Stadler *et al.*, 1991; Palmer *et al.*, 1992; Stefanovic-Racic *et al.*,
1992) a response attributed to iNOS. Cytokines have also been shown to induce NO
production in human articular chondrocytes, synoviocytes and also, arguably, in
articular osteoblasts and synovial fibroblasts (Rediske *et al.*, 1994; Sakurai *et al.*,
1995; Grabowski *et al.*, 1996). By immunohistochemical and *in situ* hybridization
analyses of synovial and cartilage tissue from RA patients, Sakurai and colleagues
further reported strong iNOS expression in synoviocytes, endothelial cells, chondrocytes, and, to a lesser extent, synovial fibroblasts (Chapter 5). Similar findings
were published by McInnes *et al.* (1996). In addition to these joint-derived cells,
iNOS induced in mast cells and infiltrating macrophages, neutrophils and lymphocytes probably also contributes to the increased intra-articular NO production in
joint inflammation (reviewed by Evans and Stefanovic-Racic (1996)). These
putative sites for NO generation in the joint are illustrated in Figure 4.1.

4.3 Regulation of synovial blood flow

The nutritional requirements of avascular structures such as cartilage within the
joint are supplied by synovial fluid, the production of which is dependent on blood
flow to the joint. The factors regulating synovial blood flow, therefore, play an
essential role in maintaining the integrity of diathroidal joints, yet they remain
incompletely understood. Neural influences are known to contribute a dominant
component to this regulation: sympathetic post-ganglionic fibres innervating the
knee joint mediate vasoconstrictor 'tone' (see below), and articular sensory nerves
release vasodilating neuropeptides from their peripheral terminals in the synovium
(see below). Prostaglandins also contribute as vasodilators to the regulation of the
joint vasculature, since indomethacin infusion was found to reduce basal blood

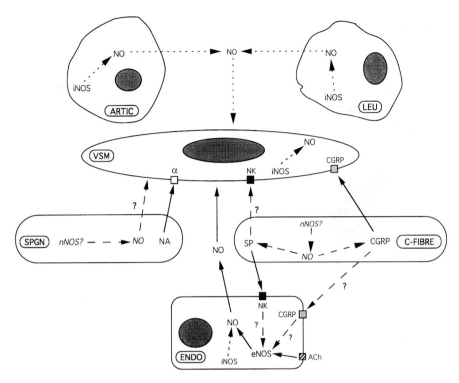

Figure 4.1. Schematic diagram of known and potential sources of NO acting on vascular smooth muscle (VSM) in the synovium, including possible locations of NOS. ARTIC, articular cells (e.g. fibroblasts, synoviocytes, chondrocytes, mast cells); ENDO, endothelial cell; LEU, leukocyte (e.g. macrophages, neutrophils, lymphocytes); SPGN, sympathetic post-ganglionic neurone; C-FIBRE, unmyelinated sensory afferent nerve terminal; NA, noradrenaline; SP, substance P, CGRP, calcitonin gene-related peptide; NK, tachykinin (neurokinin) receptor, α, α-adrenoceptor; ACh, acetylcholine. Italicized lettering and dashed lines accompanied by (?) indicate hypothesized pathways. Dotted lines indicate induced pathways.

flow in the rabbit knee (Najafipour and Ferrell, 1994). They appear, however, to have little influence on modulating sympathetic vasoconstrictor responses. Angiotensin II, a potent vasoconstrictor of peripheral vascular beds, may also serve a paracrine role in regulating synovial blood flow, since local generation of angiotensin II in the joint is implicated by the detection of angiotensin-converting enzyme (Walsh *et al.*, 1993) and angiotensin AT1 receptors (Walsh *et al.*, 1994) in the human synovium.

More recently, it has become appreciated that NO also plays an important role in regulating synovial perfusion in the normal joint. Evidence for tonic release of NO is provided by the finding that close intra-arterial infusion of L-NAME (N^w-nitro-L-arginine methylester; 3 mg/kg per h) produced a substantial ($\sim 100\%$) increase in resistance in the rabbit knee joint vasculature, which could be significantly reversed by subsequent infusion of L-arginine (Najafipour and Ferrell, 1993). In a previous study in rats, we reported only an initial 15% increase in joint vascular resistance with L-NAME infused intravenously (i.v.) at 1 mg/kg per h (McDougall and Ferrell, 1996), although more recent pilot work has found that bolus i.v. injections of 10 mg/kg L-NAME in rats can significantly increase vascular resistance in the knee joint by nearly 100% ($P = 0.009$, $n = 7$; unpublished observations). Also in the rat, other investigators have reported that ^{133}Xe clearance from the synovial cavity was reduced nearly 40% by 0.1 μmol bolus injections of L-NAME into the joint (Cambridge and Brain, 1995), a finding consistent with basal release of NO contributing to the regulation of joint perfusion.

Tonic release of NO also occurs in inflamed joints, as demonstrated in an acute model of arthritis (Najafipour and Ferrell, 1993). This model is induced by intra-articular injection of carrageenan, which results in an acute inflammatory response that is fully developed by 24 h and is characterized by synovial infiltration of polymorphonuclear leukocytes. As in the normal, non-inflamed, rabbit knee, close intra-arterial infusion of L-NAME was found to cause a fall in synovial perfusion in the carrageenan-inflamed rabbit knee, although the change in vascular resistance tended to be smaller (69% increase) than in the normal joint. While one interpretation of this finding could be that NO does not contribute to inflammatory hyperaemia, it is important to recognize that L-NAME is considered to be more effective at inhibiting eNOS than the iNOS isoform (Rees et al., 1990; McCall et al., 1991). As any difference in the amount of NO generated in the normal compared with the carrageenan-injected knee is probably the result of a greater activity of iNOS in the latter, future studies with specific NOS inhibitors would be useful to establish whether NO contributes to the hyperaemia associated with joint inflammation. From a therapeutic viewpoint, it would be valuable for such studies to investigate whether selective inhibition of iNOS could suppress inflammatory hyperaemia without undermining the physiological role of NO in regulating synovial perfusion, since the latter is essential for the maintenance of the functional integrity of the joint. To date, no studies have examined whether the tonic release of NO and its effects on basal synovial perfusion are altered in more chronic models of joint inflammation.

The contribution of NO to the regulation of synovial blood flow may, in part, involve interaction with substance P and calcitonin gene-related peptide (CGRP). These neuropeptides are coreleased in the knee joint from the peripheral terminals of sensory nerves and have been shown to increase synovial blood flow (Lam and Ferrell, 1993a). In recent work, we have suggested that the tonic release of endogenous substance P and CGRP may in fact be partly responsible for main-tenance of synovial blood flow, since separately administering specific antagonists for each of these neuropeptides resulted in a significant fall in basal perfusion of the synovium (Karimian and Ferrell, 1996; McMurdo, Lockhart and Ferrell, 1996; see Figure 4.2). This is relevant to the present discussion since there is evidence in the literature that the vasoactive effects of substance P (Whittle, Lopez-Belmonte and Rees, 1989) and CGRP (Chen and Guth, 1995) may be at least partially NO dependent, although other groups have suggested NO may be important for the

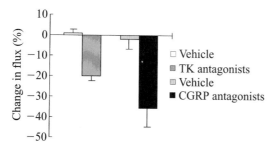

Figure 4.2. Changes in blood flow (flux) of the rat knee joint in response to combined administration of the tachykinin (TK) NK_1 receptor antagonist FK888 and the tachykinin NK_2 receptor antagonist SR48968 (both 10^{-8} mol) or administration of the CGRP receptor antagonist $CGRP_{(8-37)}$ (1.5×10^{-9} mol, topical), and their respective vehicles. Blood flow was measured by laser Doppler perfusion imaging. Data are expressed as mean $\pm$S.E. mean for five or six observations. $^{*}P < 0.05$ when compared with vehicle control.

release but not actions of neuropeptides in the skin (Holzer and Jocic, 1994; Kajekar *et al.*, 1995). Whether NO facilitates neuropeptide release in the joint or acts to mediate its vasorelaxant effects on the synovial vasculature has yet to be established.

From *in vitro* studies on rabbit articular chondrocytes (Stadler *et al.*, 1991), NO is also known to interact with COX, the enzyme responsible for synthesizing prostaglandins from arachidonic acid. The manner of this interaction, however, appears to depend on the concentration of NO, since low levels increased prostaglandin E_2 production whereas high levels of NO caused a decrease. Although changes were not studied specifically in the joint, Salvemini and colleagues have since extended this work *in vivo* by administering NO exogenously to rats. They found that i.v. injection of NO donors enhanced prostaglandin formation, presumably via stimulation of the constitutive form of the endogenous COX enzyme (Salvemini and Masferrer, 1996; Chapter 7). Since, as stated above, prostaglandins act to vasodilate synovial vessels, it is conceivable that NO may act to increase joint blood flow partly via the stimulation of prostaglandin production. The interaction of these two systems, particularly during acute and chronic joint inflammation, merits further investigation.

4.4 NO modulation of sympathetic-mediated vasocontriction

In all species examined to date, electrical stimulation of nerves supplying the knee joint elicits a frequency-dependent vasoconstriction mediated by the adrenergic neurotransmitter, noradrenaline (Lam and Ferell, 1993b; Karimian, McDougall and Ferell, 1995). Moreover, sympathetic post-ganglionic fibres innervating the joint contribute to the vasoconstrictor 'tone' exhibited by articular blood vessels (Cobbold and Lewis, 1956; Koshbaten and Ferrell, 1990). Evidence that this nerve-mediated vasoconstriction is modulated by NO is provided by the work of

Najafipour and Ferrell (1993), in which they demonstrated that L-NAME infusion in the rabbit increased the magnitude of the vasoconstrictor response both to electrical stimulation of the nerve supply to the joint and to intra-arterial injection of α-adrenoceptor agonists.

There is, however, species variation in the magnitude of the effect of inhibiting NO synthesis on nerve-mediated vasoconstriction. While L-NAME administration in the rabbit enhances the constrictor response to nerve stimulation at 30 Hz by approximately 70%, the same stimulus parameters in rats elicited as much as a threefold increase in the constrictor response when NO synthesis was inhibited using another inhibitor of NOS, L-NMMA (McDougall and Ferrell, 1996). In fact, inhibiting NO both increased the basal vascular resistance and enhanced the nerve-mediated constrictor response by a similar magnitude in the rabbit ($\sim$ 70%), whereas in the rat the basal resistance changed little compared with the over 300% change in the constrictor reponse. This could reflect additional NO release in response to electrical stimulation from peripheral nerve terminals present in the rat joint.

A neural source for NO in the rat joint is also implicated by the observation that while the frequency-dependent vasoconstriction elicited by nerve stimulation was considerably enhanced by L-NMMA, L-NAME failed to elicit such an effect even when infused at a dose producing a comparable rise in arterial blood pressure (McDougall and Ferrell, 1996). A possible explanation for this intriguing difference could again lie with the relative affinities of L-NMMA and L-NAME for the different isoforms of NOS. L-NMMA is believed to inhibit all the NOS isoforms (Rees *et al.*, 1990), whereas L-NAME, although still relatively non-selective, may at the concentration used in these studies have had a greater inhibitory effect on the endothelial form of the enzyme than on either the neural or inducible isoforms. As the joints were not inflamed, iNOS is unlikely to have been present in significant quantities. The differential action of L-NMMA and L-NAME could, therefore, suggest that nNOS is present in nerves supplying the synovium. Development of specific inhibitors for the different isoforms of NOS may now allow this issue to be clarified. Further investigation is also required to elucidate which of the nerve types innervating the joint might serve as a source for neurally derived NO. In addition to the sympathetic efferent fibres, potential candidates include the large myelinated afferent fibres, which serve primarily a proprioceptive function, and the more populous unmyelinated and finely myelinated axons associated with neuropeptide release.

Acute joint inflammation reduces the magnitude of nerve-mediated constrictor responses in both rabbits (Najafipour and Ferrell, 1993) and rats (Lam and Ferrell, 1993b). However, this effect is probably a consequence of impaired sympathetic neurotransmission, since close intra-arterial injection of α-adrenoceptor agonists at single doses in the rabbit revealed no significant differences between normal and inflamed knees (Najafipour and Ferrell, 1993). Similarly in the rat knee joint, topical application of noradrenaline elicits dose-dependent vasoconstriction that is unaffected by acute joint inflammation (Figure 4.3).

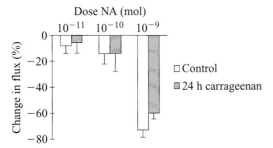

Figure 4.3. Nonadrenaline (NA, topical) elicits a dose-dependent decrease in blood flow (flux) to the rat knee joint as measured by laser Doppler perfusion imaging. This response to noradrenaline is unaltered in rats 24 h after intra-articular injection of 2% carrageenan. Data are expressed as mean ±S.E. mean for seven or eight observations.

4.5 Effects of inflammation on synovial reactivity

The reactivity of the synovial vasculature can be assessed by exogenous administration of vasoactive agents to the joint. Acetylcholine is known to induce an endothelium-dependent vasodilatation via release of NO in many vascular beds, and our ongoing research suggests this is also true in the rabbit knee joint vasculature (Figure 4.4). The vasodilator effect of acetylcholine (10 nmol) given as close intra-arterial bolus injections is considerably reduced by i.v. infusion of L-NAME at 12 mg/kg per h and partially restored by L-arginine (240 mg/kg per h). However, we find that the vascular reactivity to acetylcholine is much diminished ($P < 0.001$) in the acutely inflamed rabbit knee studied 24 h after carrageenan injection, with infusions of L-NAME and L-arginine having minimal effect on this suppressed vasodilator response to acetylcholine. This altered reactivity suggests that the vascular endothelial function of the synovium may be undermined or that the sensitivity of the synovial vasculature diminished during acute inflammation in the rabbit.

Close intra-arterial injection of acetylcholine also dilates the vasculature of the rat knee joint, as illustrated in the perfusion scans obtained from a laser Doppler imager (Figure 4.5). This recently developed technique generates a two-dimensional spatial perfusion map of a scanned area and has been validated in our laboratory for assessing joint perfusion by comparison with absolute blood flow measurements obtained using radiolabelled microspheres ($r = 0.94$, $P = 0.006$, $n = 6$). In ongoing studies, we find topical application of 10 nmol acetylcholine to the exposed rat knee similarly induces a vasodilator response, although this response, unlike in the rabbit, is significantly enhanced in the carrageenan-inflamed joint (Figure 4.6(a)). While the NO-dependence of this response has not yet been investigated using an inhibitor of NO synthesis, sodium nitroprusside was also administered topically to the knees in these experiments. This NO donor acts independently of the endothelium and was found to yield a similar magnitude of vasodilatation in both the normal and inflamed joint. Therefore, the enhanced effect of acetylcholine during acute inflammation in the rat is probably an endothelium-mediated effect.

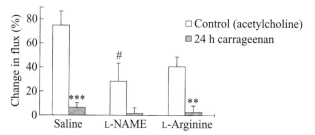

Figure 4.4. Changes in blood flow (flux) of the rabbit knee joint in response to acetylcholine (10^{-8} mol, close intra-arterial injection) as measured by laser Doppler perfusion imaging. Acetylcholine elicits an increase in flux that is significantly attenuated in rabbits treated with L-NAME (12 mg/kg per h i.v.) and partially restored by L-arginine (240 mg/kg per h) (open columns). The acetylcholine-induced vasodilatation is significantly reduced in rabbits given carrageenan (2%; intra-articular) 24 h prior to acetylcholine administration, an effect that is unaltered by application of either L-NAME or L-arginine (hatched columns). Data are expressed as mean ±S.E. mean for four or five observations. $**P<0.01$, $***P<0.001$ when compared with control/non-inflamed knees. $^{\#}P<0.05$ when compared with saline control.

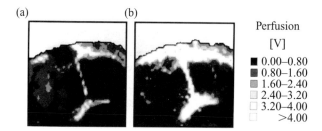

Figure 4.5. Laser Doppler perfusion images of the medial aspect of the exposed rat knee, before (a) and after (b) topical application of acetylcholine (0.1 μmol). The images are coded in grey-scale with highest perfusion represented in white and lowest perfusion in black. Note the increase in perfusion in the area of the synovium (upper region of b) with acetylcholine. The area of high perfusion in the lower region of the images is attributable to the saphenous vessels. Note also the collateral supplying the synovial region from these vessels.

We are currently investigating the mechanisms responsible for the differential effects of acute inflammation in rat and rabbit on the synovial vascular reactivity to acetylcholine.

Interestingly, NO-mediated vasoregulation also appears to be altered in more chronic models of joint inflammation. For instance, McDougall, Karimian and Ferrell (1995) demonstrated that substance P-induced vasodilatation in the rat joint vasculature was completely abolished in an adjuvant model of arthritis. This is of relevance since substance P-mediated vasorelaxation is thought to be at least partially NO dependent (Whittle *et al.*, 1989). More recent work from our laboratory has found that the vasodilator response to acetylcholine is reduced by as much as 54% in this rat model of arthritis (Figure 4.6(b)). Taken together, these findings suggest that NO-mediated vasorelaxation in the synovium is substantially,

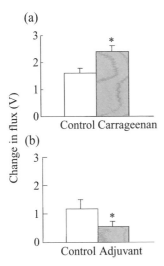

Figure 4.6. Changes in blood flow (flux) of the rat knee joint in response to acetylcholine (10^{-8} mol, topical) measured by laser Doppler perfusion imaging. (a) Acetylcholine elicits an increase in flux in control rats that is significantly enhanced in rats pre-treated (24 h) with 0.1 ml carrageenan (2%; intra-articular). (b) Acetylcholine elicits an increase in flux in control rats that is significantly attenuated in rats pre-treated (7 days) with Freund's complete adjuvant (0.2 mg; intra-articular). Data are expressed as mean $\pm$S.E. mean for six or seven observations. $^{*}P < 0.05$ when compared with vehicle control.

if not completely, abolished in the arthritic joint. The reasons for this are not yet known, although one explanation could be that an enhancement in the levels of NO within the synovial cavity may cause tachykinin and cholinergic receptor down-regulation. Another explanation could be that the endothelium/receptor-transduction mechanisms have been damaged in this chronic model of joint inflammation; alternatively, the synovial vasculature could be already maximally vasodilated and, therefore, unresponsive to exogenous application of vasodilators such as substance P or acetylcholine. Again, elucidation of the mechanisms for this altered vascular reactivity requires further experimental work.

4.6 Conclusions

From these studies, it may be concluded that NO fulfils an important function as a vasodilator in the regulation of blood flow in joints. The relative contribution of various cell types in the joint capsule to intra-articular generation of NO is incompletely understood (Figure 4.1), but is likely to include constitutively pro-duced NO from vascular endothelial cells and possibly also from nerves innervating the joint. In addition, NO induced during joint inflammation from articular cells and invading leukocytes probably contributes to the increased synovial fluid concentrations of NO in arthritis. NO is also important for the vascular reactivity of the synovial vasculature to sympathetic nerve stimulation and exogenous administration of acetylcholine, although the nature of this role is altered during acute and chronic joint inflammation and varies depending on the species studied. As synovial joints are important sites of acute and chronic inflammation, possible conflict may arise between the roles for NO in the regulation of normal joint blood flow and in the arthritic inflammatory processes. Consequently, the recent development of selective iNOS inhibitors could have therapeutic value in suppressing inflammatory hyperaemia without undermining normal joint perfusion. Clearly much still remains to be investigated regarding the regulation of joint blood flow by NO, and the relevance of this to the pathogenesis and progression of arthritis.

Acknowledgements

The authors acknowledge the contributions of Dr W. J. Angerson and Miss S. Young who participated in some of the experiments presented in the text. Expert technical assistance was provided by Mrs H. Collin. Our research is supported by the MacFeat Bequest of the University of Glasgow, and the Arthritis and Rheumatism Council.

References

Arend, W. P. and Dayer, J.-M. (1990) Cytokines and cytokine induced inhibitors or agonists in rheumatoid arthritis. *Arthritis Rheum.* **33**, 305.

Bredt, D. S., Hwang, P. M. and Snyder, S. H. (1990) Localization of nitric oxide synthase indicating a neural role for nitric oxide. *Nature* **347**, 768–770.

Cambridge, H. and Brain, S. D. (1995) Mechanism of bradykinin-induced plasma extravasation in the rat knee joint. *Br. J. Pharmacol.* **115**, 641–647.

Chen, R. Y. Z. and Guth, P. H. (1995) Interaction of endogenous nitric oxide and CGRP in sensory neuron-induced gastric vasodilation. *Am. J. Physiol.* **268**, G791–G796.

Cobbold, A. F. and Lewis, O. J. (1956) The nervous control of joint blood vessels. *J. Physiol. (Lond.)* **133**, 467–471.

Connor, J. R., Manning, P. T., Settle, S. L. *et al.* (1995) Suppression of adjuvant-induced arthritis by selective inhibition of inducible nitric oxide synthase. *Eur. J. Pharmacol.* **273**, 15–24.

Evans, C. H. and Stefanovic-Racic, M. (1996) Nitric oxide and arthritis. *Methods: Comp. Meth. Enzymol.* **10**, 38–42.

Farrell, A. J., Blake, D. R., Palmer, R. M. J. and Moncada, S. (1992) Increased concentrations of nitrite in synovial fluid and serum samples suggest increased nitric oxide synthesis in rheumatic diseases. *Ann. Rheumat. Dis.* **51**, 1219–1222.

Grabowski, P. S., Macpherson, H. and Ralston, S. H. (1996) Nitric oxide production in cells derived from the human joint. *Br. J. Rheumatol.* **35**, 207–212.

Grozdanovic, Z., Bruning, G. and Baumgarten, H. G. (1994) Nitric oxide – a novel autonomic neurotransmitter. *Acta Anatom.* **150**, 16–24.

Holzer, P. and Jocic, M. (1994) Cutaneous vasodilation induced by nitric oxide-evoked stimulation of afferent nerves in the rat. *Br. J. Pharmacol.* **112**, 1181–1187.

Ialenti, A., Moncada, S. and Di Rosa, M. (1993) Modulation of adjuvant arthritis by endogenous nitric oxide. *Br. J. Pharmacol.* **110**, 701–706.

Ignarro, L. J., Buga, G. M., Wood, K. S., Byrns, R. E. and Chaudhuri, G. (1987) Endothelium-derived relaxing factor produced and released from artery and vein is nitric oxide. *Proc. Nat. Acad. Sci. USA* **84**, 9265–9269.

Kajekar, R., Moore, P. K. and Brain, S. D. (1995) Essential role for nitric oxide in neurogenic inflammation in rat cutaneous microcirculation: evidence for an endothelium-independent mechansim. *Circ. Res.* **76**, 441–447.

Karimian, S. M. and Ferrell, W. R. (1996) Tachykinin modulation of synovial blood flow. *J. Autonom. Nerv. Syst.* **58**, 211–212.

Karimian, S. M., McDougall, J. J. and Ferrell, W. R. (1995) Neuropeptidergic and autonomic control of the vasculature of the rat knee joint revealed by laser Doppler perfusion imaging. *Exp. Physiol.* **80**, 341–348.

Knowles, R. G. and Moncada, S. (1994) Nitric oxide synthases in mammals. *Biochem. J.* **298**, 249–258.

Koshbaten, A. and Ferrell, W. R. (1990) Alterations in cat knee joint blood flow induced by electrical stimulation of articular afferents and efferents. *J. Physiol. (Lond.)* **430**, 77–86.

Lam, F. Y. and Ferrell, W. R. (1993a) Effects of interactions of naturally-occurring neuro-peptides on blood flow in the rat knee joint. *Br. J. Pharmacol.* **108**, 694–699.

Lam, F. Y. and Ferrell, W. R. (1993b) Acute inflammation in the rat knee joint attenuates sympathetic vasoconstriction but enhances neuropeptide-mediated vasodilatation assessed by laser Doppler perfusion imaging. *Neuroscience* **52**, 443–449.

McCall, T. B., Feelisch, M., Palmer, R. M. J. and Moncada, S. (1991) Identification of *N*-iminoethyl-L-ornithine as an irreversible inhibitor of nitric oxide synthase in phagocytic cells. *Br. J. Pharmacol.* **102**, 234–238.

McCartney-Francis, N., Allen, J. B., Mitzel, D. E. *et al.* (1993) Suppression of arthritis by an inhibitor of nitric oxide sythase. *J. Exp. Med.* **178**, 749–754.

McDougall, J. J. and Ferrell, W. R. (1996) Inhibition of nitric oxide production during electrical stimulation of the nerves supplying the rat knee joint. *J. Autonom. Nerv. Syst.* **57**, 73–77.

McDougall, J. J., Karimian, S. M. and Ferrell, W. R. (1995) Prolonged alteration of vasoconstrictor and vasodilator responses in rat knee joints by adjuvant monoarthritis. *Exp. Physiol.* **80**, 349–357.

McInnes, I. B., Leung, B. P., Field, M. *et al.* (1996) Production of nitric oxide in the synovial membrane of rheumatoid and osteoarthritis patients. *J. Exp. Med.* **184**, 1519–1524.

McMurdo, L., Lockhart, J. C. and Ferrell, W. R. (1996) Modulation of rat synovial blood flow by the CGRP receptor antagonist, CGRP(8–37). *Br. J. Pharmacol.* **119**, 82P.

Najafipour, H. and Ferrell, W. R. (1993) Nitric oxide modulates sympathetic vasoconstriction and basal blood flow in normal and acutely inflamed rabbit knee joints. *Exp. Physiol.* **78**, 615–624.

Najafipour, H. and Ferrell, W. R. (1994) Role of prostaglandins in regulation of blood flow and modulation of sympathetic vasoconstriction in normal and acutely inflamed rabbit knee joints. *Exp. Physiol.* **79**, 93–101.

Palmer, R. M. J., Andrews, T., Foxwell, N. A. and Moncada, S. (1992) Glucocorticoids do not affect the induction of a novel calcium-dependent nitric oxide synthase in rabbit chondrocytes. *Biochem. Biophys. Res. Commun.* **188**, 209–215.

Rediske, J. J., Koehne, C. F., Zhang, B. and Lotz, M. (1994) The inducible production of nitric oxide by articular cell types. *Osteoarthritis and Cartilage* **2**, 199–206.

Rees, D. D., Palmer, R. M. J., Schulz, R., Hodson, H. F. and Moncada, S. (1990) Characterisation of three inhibitors of endothelial nitric oxide synthase *in vitro* and *in vivo*. *Br. J. Pharmacol.* **101**, 746–752.

Sakurai, H., Kohsaka, H., Lui, M.-F. *et al.* (1995) Nitric oxide production and inducible nitric oxide synthase expression in inflammatory arthritides. *J. Clin. Invest.* **96**, 2357–2363.

Salvemini, D. and Masferrer, J. L. (1996) Interation of nitric oxide with cyclooxygenase: *in vitro*, *ex vivo* and *in vivo* studies. *Meth. Enzymol.* **269**, 12–25.

Stadler, J., Stefanovic-Racic, M., Billiar, T. R. *et al.* (1991) Articular chondrocytes synthesize nitric oxide in response to cytokines and lipopolysaccharide. *J. Immunol.* **147**, 3915–3920.

Stefanovic-Racic, M., Stadler, J., Feorgescu, H. I. and Evans, C. H. (1992) Nitric oxide production by cytokine stimulated synovial fibroblasts. *Trans. Orthapaed. Res. Soc.* **17**, 228.

Stefanovic-Racic, M., Meyers, K., Meschter, C., Coffey, J. W., Hoffman, R. A. and Evans, C. H. (1994) *N*-Monomethyl arginine, an inhibitor of nitric oxide synthase, suppresses the development of adjuvant arthritis in rats. *Arthritis Rheum.* **37**, 1062–1069.

Ueki, Y., Miyake, S., Tominaga, Y. and Eguchi, K. (1996) Increased nitric oxide levels in patients with rheumatoid arthritis. *J. Rheumatol.* **23**, 230–236.

Walsh, D. A., Mapp, P. I., Wharton, J., Polak, J. M. and Blake, D. R. (1993) Neuropeptide degrading enzymes in normal and inflamed human synovium. *Am. J. Pathol.* **142**, 1610–1621.

Walsh, D. A., Suzuki, T., Knock, G. A., Blake, D. R., Polak, J. M. and Wharton, J. (1994) AT₁ receptor characteristics of angiotensin analogue binding in human synovium. *Br. J. Pharmacol.* **112**, 435–442.

Whittle, B. J. R., Lopez-Belmonte, J. and Rees, D. D. (1989) Modulation of the vasodepressor actions of acetylcholine, bradykinin, substance P and endothelin in the rat by a specific inhibitor of nitric oxide formation. *Br. J. Pharmacol.* **98**, 646–652.

5

Nitric oxide production in human inflammatory arthritides

NOBUYUKI MIYASAKA and YUKIO HIRATA

5.1 Introduction

Inducible NOS expression and NO synthesis have been characterized in several rodent *in vivo* models of organ-specific autoimmune diseases, such as experimental allergic encephalomyelitis (EAE) (Cross *et al.*, 1993) and immunologically induced diabetes in non-obese diabetic (NOD) mice (Corbett *et al.* 1993). Furthermore, augmented NO production and iNOS expression have been reported in several animal models of arthritis including MRL/*1pr* mice (Weinburg *et al.*, 1994), streptococcal cell-wall fragment model (McCartney-Francis *et al.*, 1993), adjuvant-induced arthritis (Stefanovic-Racic *et al.*, 1994) and collagen-induced arthritis (Cannon *et al.*, 1996). The onset of arthritis was blocked by the NOS inhibitor L-NMMA, suggesting that NO might play an important role in the induction maintenance of arthritis in these models.

RA is a human autoimmune disease characterized by chronic inflammation of the synovial tissues in multiple joints. It causes also extraarticular manifestations such as interstitial pneumonitis and vasculitis. Pathologically, it is characterized by intense infiltration of T cells and macrophages, marked hyperplasia of synovial lining cells and neovascularization of the synovium. Infiltrating T cells are predominantly CD4$^+$/CD45RO$^+$ cells expressing various activation markers including HLA-DR molecules. Activation of monocytes/macrophages is also marked, as shown by abundant production of inflammatory cytokines, such as IL-1, IL-6, TNFα, and GM-CSF (Feldmann, Brennan and Maini, 1996), and of multiple low-molecular-weight bioactive substances, including endothelin-1, a potent vasoconstrictive peptide (Miyasaka *et al.*, 1992). Synovial macrophages surrounding T cell foci express costimulatory molecules such as CD86 and CD40, contributing to the sustained immune responses between infiltrating T cells and synovial cells in patients with RA (Liu *et al.*, 1996; Sekine *et al.*, 1998).

In this chapter, we describe excessive NO production and iNOS expression in various compartments of human inflammatory athritides, including RA, and discuss their pathophysiological significance in these disorders.

5.2 Urinary NO metabolite excretion

A major source of urinary nitrate is endogenously synthesized NO if there is no excess dietary intake of nitrite. NO is rapidly oxidized to nitrite and nitrate and excreted into the urine. Urinary nitrate excretion in RA patients was 2.7-fold greater than that in healthy controls and was reduced by the administration of prednisolone (Stichtenoth *et al.*, 1995). However, the amount of urinary nitrate excretion did not correlate with values of C-reactive protein (CRP), erythrocyte sedimentation rate, joint count or duration of morning stiffness. Urinary nitrate: creatinine ratios are also reported to be significantly elavated (average threefold elevation) in RA patients (Grabowski *et al.*, 1996). These studies indicate excessive *in vivo* NO sythesis in RA patients.

5.3 Serum NO metabolite levels

Serum nitrite concentrations in patients with RA and osteoarthritis were significantly higher than in age- and sex- matched controls (Farrell *et al.*, 1992). Serum nitrite concentration in RA was higher than that in osteoarthritis, which may reflect the intense inflammatory changes in RA. However, there was no significant correlation between serum nitrite and CRP. This could also be explained by the timing of blood sampling, as nitrite has a short serum half life.

Levels of 3-nitrotyrosine, which can be produced by NO-dependent oxidative damage, are also elevated in patients with active RA (Kaur and Halliwell, 1994). In contrast, sera from osteoarthritic patients and normal controls had no detectable 3-nitrotyrosine using HPLC analysis. A recent study using a sensitive chemiluminescence assay indicated that serum NO metabolite levels were higher in patients with RA than in patients with osteoarthritis or in healthy subjects (Ueki *et al.*, 1996). Furthermore, NO levels correlated with the disease activity when assessed by duration of morning stiffness, the number of tender or swollen joints and CRP in the same study. NO metabolite levels also significantly correlated with those of TNFα and IL-6 in RA sera. These studies suggest that up-regulated NO metabolite in sera of RA patients may reflect heightened inflammatory changes in the joint.

5.4 NO production by peripheral blood mononuclear cells

A recent report showed that peripheral blood mononuclear cells from RA patients had increased iNOS activity compared with those from normal controls, thus indicating also a systemic activation of the iNOS protein in RA patients (St Clair *et al.*, 1996). Stimulation of mononuclear cells with IFN-γ resulted in increased iNOS expression and nitrite/nitrate production *in vitro*. iNOS activity of mononuclear cells correlated with the disease activity, as assessed by tender and swollen joint counts.

5.5 Synovial fluid NO metabolite levels

Synovial fluid nitrite has been shown to be significantly higher than serum nitrite in patients with RA, indicating local NO synthesis in rheumatoid joints (Farrell *et al.*, 1992). Nitrotyrosine has also been shown to be increased in synovial fluid from patients with RA (Kaur and Halliwell, 1994). Our group and others have found that NO metabolites are increased not only in patients with RA but also in patients with osteoarthritis or gout; therefore, we speculate that increased NO production is not unique to RA but rather may reflect non-specific inflammatory changes, though not necessarily specific immune responses in the lesions (Farrell *et al.*, 1992; Sakurai *et al.*, 1995).

5.6 NO production by synovial tissue

Ex-vivo cultured rheumatoid synovium and chondrocytes produce a significant amount of nitrite, and the addition of L-NMMA to the culture inhibits this nitrite production (Figure 5.1) (Sakurai *et al.*, 1995). Immunohistochemical studies and *in situ* hybridization analysis have revealed that both the iNOS protein and its mRNA are predominantly expressed in synovial lining cells, endothelial cells, chondrocytes and, to a lesser extent, the infiltrating mononuclear cells and synovial fibroblasts (Figure 5.2). Most of the synovial lining cells and infiltrating mononuclear cells immunoreactive to iNOS express CD14 and HLA-DR, which suggests that most of iNOS producing cells are type A synovial cells. Normal synovium expressed iNOS protein minimally in both the lining and endothelium. Western blot analysis of rheumatoid synovial cells showed the presence of a 130 kDa protein corresponding to the authentic human iNOS protein. Reverse transcriptase (RT) polymerase chain reaction (PCR) analysis also confirmed an abundant iNOS mRNA expression in

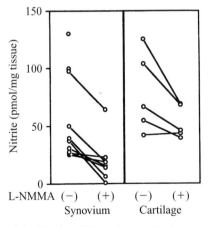

Figure 5.1. *Ex vivo* NO production by the synovium and the cartilage from RA patients and its inhibition by L-NMMA. A 50 mg synovium or cartilage sample was cultured for 24 h in the presence or absence of 0.5 mM L-NMMA. The nitrite concentration in the culture medium was assayed by the Griess reaction.

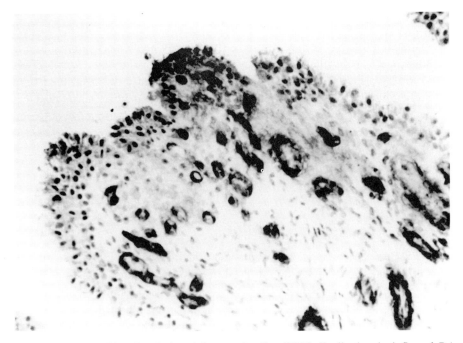

Figure 5.2. Immunohistochemical staining to visualize iNOS distribution in inflamed RA synovium. iNOS was found to be expressed by synovial lining cells, endothelial cells, some infiltrating cells and fibroblasts ($\times 100$).

both RA and osteoarthritic synovium (Figure 5.3). NO production by freshly iso-lated synovial cells was up-regulated by stimulation with a combination of IL-1β, TNFα and LPS (Figure 5.4). However, synovial fibroblast cell lines in long-term culture did not liberate NO even after stimulation. In this connection, others recently reported that most of the iNOS-producing synovial cells in both RA and osteoarthritic synovium are negative for non-specific esterase (NSE) and CD68, which are thought to be macrophage markers; only a minor population immuno-reactive to iNOS expressed both markers (McInnes *et al.*, 1996). These authors speculate that the majority of iNOS-producing cells among synovial cells are synovial fibroblasts (synovial B cells). They also showed that synovial adherent cells stimulated with *S*-nitroso-acetylpenicillamine, an NO donor, produced high concentrations of TNFα in the culture.

5.7 Significance of NO production in rheumatoid arthritis

Whether excessive NO production in RA is proinflammatory or anti-inflammatory remains to be clarified. Possible proinflammatory effects of NO include augmenta-tion of vascular permeability in inflamed tissues (Mayhan, 1992), generation of destructive free radicals such as the peroxynitrite and hydroxyl radicals (Beckman, 1990), and induction of COX-2 and inflammatory cytokines such as TNFα and IL-1 (Lander *et al.*, 1993; McInnes *et al.*, 1996). NO can also be involved in the

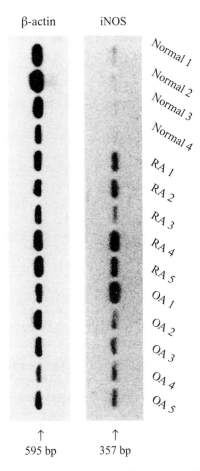

β-actin   iNOS

Normal 1
Normal 2
Normal 3
Normal 4
RA 1
RA 2
RA 3
RA 4
RA 5
OA 1
OA 2
OA 3
OA 4
OA 5

↑   ↑
595 bp   357 bp

Figure 5.3. Southern blot hybridization of iNOS RT-PCR products amplified from synovium from patients with RA and osteoarthritis. Normal 1–4, non-inflamed synovium from patients with trauma; RA 1–5, RA synovium; OA 1–5, osteoarthritic OA synovium. The iNOS mRNA was increased in inflamed synovium compared with non-inflamed synovium.

production of angiogenic cytokines (Leibovich *et al.*, 1994) and activation of matrix metalloproteases. Experimentally induced arthritis has been shown to be reversed by NOS inhibitors (McCartney-Francis *et al.*, 1993; Stefanovic-Racic *et al.*, 1994; Connor *et al.*, 1995) and mice lacking the iNOS gene show reduced non-specific inflammatory response to carrageenan (Wei *et al.*, 1995). These findings establish the crucial role of NO as an inflammatory mediator. In contrast, NO and its derivative *S*-nitrosoglutathione inhibit DNA synthesis of T cells in association with intracellular cGMP accumulation, which may explain suppressed T cell function in RA patients; therefore, NO may exert an anti-inflammatory effect in this sense (Merryman *et al.*, 1993). NO may have bi-phasic or opposite biological effects in the joints, depending on its local concentration; NO is, therefore, possibly a 'double-edged sword' in human inflammatory arthritides (Stefanovic-Racic, Stadler and Evans, 1993).

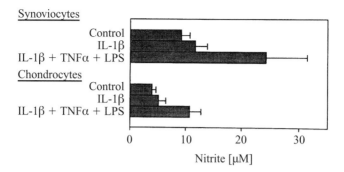

Figure 5.4. NO production from isolated rheumatoid synovial cells and chondrocytes in the presence of IL-1β alone or a combination of IL-1β, TNFα and LPS for 48 h. The nitrite in the media increased 2.5-fold by stimulation with a combination of the IL-1β, TNFα and LPS. Data are shown as means $\pm$ S.D. from triplicate cultures.

NO synthesis is under transcriptional, post-transcriptional and translational controls (Nathan and Xie, 1994). Especially cytokines such as IL-1, TNFα and IFN-γ induce NO production, whereas TGFβ and IL-10 can suppress it. These cytokines are abundantly synthesized in inflammatory synovium over a prolonged period of time (Firestein, Alvaro-Gracia and Maki, 1990) and the amount of NO present in inflamed joints could, therefore, be a net effect of the inflammatory cytokines.

NO was originally identified as EDRF, which regulates vascular tone. We have reported increased levels of endothelin-1, a potent vasoconstrictor, in inflammatory arthritides (Miyasaka et al., 1992). Endothelin-1 was shown to be mainly produced by type A synovial cells. Endothelins promote the synthesis of NO through type B receptors in vitro (Hirata et al., 1993), thus generating a possible positive feedback regulatory mechanism in inflammatory athritides. It is also intriguing to find that both vasoconstrictive and vasodilative substances are regulated in the inflammatory synovium.

5.8 Conclusions

NO is introduced as a new member of mediators overexpressed in inflammatory synovium. NO has a dual nature in inflammation; whether or not it can be therapeutic target for human arthritides including RA awaits further investigation.

References

Beckman, J. S., Beckman, T. W., Chen, T. W., Marshall, P. A. and Freeman, B. A. (1990) Apparent hydroxyl radical production by peroxynitrite: implications for endothelial injury from nitric oxide and superoxide. Proc. Natl. Acad. Sci., USA 87, 1620–1624.

Cannon, G. W., Oppenshaw, S. J., Hibbs, J. B. et al., (1996) Nitric oxide production during adjuvant-induced and collegen-induced arthritis. Arthritis Rheum. 39, 1677–1684.

Connor, J. R., Manning, P. T., Settle, S. L. *et al.*, (1995) Suppression of adjuvant-induced arthritis by selective inhibition of inducible nitric oxide synthase. *Eur. J. Pharmacol.* **273**, 15–24.

Corbett, J. A., Mikhael, A., Shimizu, J. *et al.*, (1993) Nitric oxide production in islets from nonobese diabetic mice: aminoguanidine sensitive and -resistant stages in the immunological diabetic process. *Proc. Nat. Acad. Sci. USA*, **90**, 8992–8995.

Cross, A. H., Misko, T. P., Lin, R. F. *et al.*, (1993) Aminoguanidine, an inhibitor of inducible nitric oxide synthase, ameliorates experimental autoimmune encephalomyelitis in SJL mice. *J. Clin. Invest.* **93**, 2684–2690.

Farrell, A. J., Blake, D. R., Palmer, R. M. *et al.*, (1992) Increased concentration of nitrite in synovial fluid and serum samples suggest increased nitric oxide synthesis in rheumatic diseases. *Ann. Rheum. Dis.* **51**, 1219–1222.

Feldmann, M., Brennan, F. M. and Maini, R. N. (1996) Rheumatoid arthritis. *Cell*, **85**, 307–310.

Firestein, G. S., Alvaro-Gracia, J. M. and Maki, R. (1990) Quantitative analysis of cytokine gene expression in rheumatoid arthritis. *J. Immunol.* **144**, 3347–3353.

Grabowski, P. S., England, A. J., Dykhuizen, R. *et al.*, (1996) Elevated nitric oxide production in rheumatoid arthritis. Detection using the fasting urinary nitrate: creatinine ratio. *Arthritis Rheum.* **39**, 643–647.

Hirata, Y., Emori, T., Eguchi, S. *et al.* (1993) Endothelin receptor subtype B mediates synthesis of nitric oxide by cultured bovine endothelial cells. *J. Clin. Invest.* **91**, 1367–1373.

Kaur, H. and Halliwell, B. (1994) Evidence for nitric oxide-mediated oxidative damage in chronic inflammation. Nitrotyrosine in serum and synovial fluid from rheumatoid patients. *FEBS Lett.* **350**, 9-12.

Lander, H. M., Sehajpal, P., Levine, D. M. *et al.* (1993) Activation of human peripheral blood mononuclear cells by nitric oxide-generating compounds. *J. Immunol.* **150**, 1509–1516.

Leibovich, S. J., Polverini, P. J., Jong, T. W. *et al.* (1994) Production of angiogenic activity by human monocytes requires an L-arginine/nitric oxide-synthase-dependent effector mechanism. *Proc. Nat. Acad. Sci. USA* **91**, 4190–4194.

Liu, M. F., Kohsaka, H., Sakurai, H. *et al.* (1996) The presence of costimulatory molecules CD86 and CD28 in rheumatoid arthritis synovium. *Arthritis Rheum.* **39**, 110–114.

Mayhan, W. G. (1992) Role of nitric oxide in modulating permeability of hamster cheek pouch in response to adenosine 5′-diphosphate and bradykinin. *Inflammation* **16**, 295–305.

McCartney-Francis, N., Allen, J. B., Mizel, D. E. *et al.* (1993) Suppression of arthritis by an inhibitor of nitric oxide synthase. *J. Exp. Med.* **178**, 749–754.

McInnes, I. B., Leung, B. P., Field, M. *et al.* (1996) Production of nitric oxide in the synovial membrane of rheumatoid and osteoathritis patients. *J. Exp. Med.* **184**, 1519–1524.

Merryman, P. F., Clancy, R. M., He, X. Y. *et al.* (1993) Modulation of human T cell responses by nitric oxide and its derivative, *S*-nitrosoglutathione. *Arthritis Rheum.*, **10**, 1414–1421.

Miyasaka, N., Hirata, Y., Ando, K. *et al.* (1992) Increased production of endothelin-1 in patients with inflammatory arthritides. *Arthritis Rheum.* **35**, 397–400.

Nathan, C. and Xie, Q. (1994) Regulation of biosynthesis of nitric oxide. *J. Biol. Chem.* **269**, 13725–13728.

Sakurai, H., Kohsaka, H., Liu, M. F. *et al.* (1995) Nitric oxide production and inducible nitric oxide synthase expression in inflammatory arthritides. *J. Clin. Invest.* **96**, 2357–2363.

Sekine, C., Yagita, H., Miyasaka, N. *et al.* (1998) Expression and function of CD40 in rheumatoid arthritis synovium, *J. Rheumatol.*, in press.

Stefanovic-Racic, M., Stadler, J. and Evans, C. H. (1993) Nitric oxide and arthritis. *Arthritis Rheum.* **36**, 1036–1044.

Stefanovic-Racic, M., Meyers, K., Meschter, C. *et al.* (1994) *N*-Monomethyl arginine, an inhibitor of nitric oxide synthase, suppresses the development of adjuvant arthritis in rats. *Arthritis Rheum.* **37**, 1062–1069.

St Clair, E. W., Wilkinson, W. E., Lang, T. *et al.* (1996) Increased expression of blood mononuclear cell nitric oxide synthesis type 2 in rheumatoid arthritis patients. *J. Exp. Med.* **184**, 1173–1178.

Stichtentoth, D. O., Fauler, J., Zeidler, H. *et al.* (1995) Urinary nitrate excretion is increased in patients with rheumatoid arthritis and reduced by prednisolone. *Ann. Rheum. Dis.* **54**, 820–824.

Ueki, Y., Miyake, S., Tominaga, K. *et al.* (1996) Increased nitric oxide levels in patients with rheumatoid arthritis. *J. Rheumatol.* **23**, 230–236.

Wei, X., Charles, I. G., Smith, A. *et al.* (1995) Altered immune responses in mice lacking inducible nitric oxide synthase. *Nature* **375**, 408–411.

Weinburg, J. B., Granger, D. L., Pisetsky, D. S. *et al.* (1994) The role of nitric oxide in the pathogenesis of spontaneous murine autoimmune disease: increased nitric oxide production and nitric oxide synthase expression in MRL-*lpr/lpr* mice, and reduction of spontaneous glomerulonephritis and arthritis by orally administered N^ω-monomethyl-L-arginine. *J. Exp. Med.* **179**, 651–660.

6

Effects of nitric oxide synthase inhibitors in experimental models of arthritis

CHRISTOPER H. EVANS and
MAJA STEFANOVIC-RACIC

6.1 Introduction

Ever since the first evidence of NO within the joints of patients with arthritis, there has been wide speculation that suitable inhibitors of iNOS would serve as powerful, new, anti-arthritic drugs. Indeed, several major pharmaceutical companies initiated research programmes directed towards this end. Such early enthusiasm proved misplaced, and a number of these programmes have been terminated or reduced in scale. The consequent hiatus provides a timely juncture at which to review critically the data obtained during this first burst of activity.

The present chapter reviews briefly what is known of the role of NO in arthritis, especially RA, and discusses the possibilities for putting this information to clinical use. As the title suggests, emphasis is placed upon the results of experiments where NOS inhibitors have been used in animal models of arthritis (see Stefanovic-Racic, Stadler and Evans (1993), Evans (1995), Evans and Stefanovic-Racic (1997) and Stefanovic-Racic and Evans (1997) for recent reviews).

6.2 NO production in arthritis

Numerous studies now agree that the production of NO is greatly increased in both human arthritis (Table 6.1) and animal models of arthritis (Table 6.2). Because NO has a short biological half life, it is likely that intra-articular production is necessary for it to elicit local responses within joints. The data of Farrell and co-workers (Farrell et al., 1992) and Ueki and co-workers (Ueki et al., 1996) suggest that intra-articular production indeed occurs in human joints, as levels of nitrite are higher in synovial fluid than in matched serum.

Data from the study of tissues dissected from the knee joints of rabbits suggest that articular cartilage (Stadler et al., 1991), meniscus (Cao et al., 1998), ligaments (unpublished data) and synovium (Stefanovic-Racic et al., 1994a) are all potential intra-articular sources of NO (Chapter 9). Whether these tissues are also important sources of NO in human joints is less clear. The most consistent data concern the articular cartilage, which, in humans, has been reproducibly shown to produce large amounts of NO. *Ex vivo* analysis of human articular cartilage obtained from the

Table 6.1. *Evidence for elevated NO production in human arthritis*

Parameter	Tissue	Disease	Result	Reference
Nitrate/nitrite	Synovial fluid	RA, OA	Elevated	Farrel *et al.*, 1992; Ueki *et al.*, 1996
	Serum	RA, OA	Elevated	Farrell *et al.*, 1992
	Serum	RA	Elevated	Ueki *et al.*, 1996
	Serum	OA	Unchanged	Ueki *et al.*, 1996
Nitrate	Urine	RA	Elevated	Stichtentoth *et al.*, 1995; Grabowski *et al.*, 1996a
Nitrotyrosine	Synovial fluid	RA	Present	Kaur and Halliwell, 1994
	Synovial fluid	OA	Absent	Kaur and Halliwell, 1994
iNOS mRNA, protein	Synovium, cartilage	RA, OA	Present	Sakurai *et al.*, 1995
nNOS protein	Cartilage	OA	Present	Amin *et al.*, 1995
NO production (*ex vivo*)	Cartilage	OA	Present	Amin *et al.*, 1995
	Synovial fibroblasts	RA, OA	Present	McInnes *et al.*, 1996
	Synovial macrophages, lymphocytes	RA	Absent	McInnes *et al.*, 1996
	Synovial fluid, lymphocytes	RA	Absent	Grabowski *et al.*, 1996b
iNOS protein	Blood leukocytes	RA	Present	St Clair *et al.*, 1996

OA, osteoarthritis.

Table 6.2. *Evidence for elevated NO production in animal models of arthritis*

Tissue	Species	Model	Reference
Synovium	Rat	Streptococcal cell wall	McCartney-Francis et al., 1993
Peritoneal macrophages	Rat	Adjuvant	Ialenti et al., 1993
Blood	Rat	Adjuvant	Connor et al., 1995
	Mouse	K_3CrO_8	Miesel, Kurpisz and Kroger, 1996
	Mouse	Septic arthritis	Sakiniene et al., 1996
Urine	Rat	Adjuvant	Cannon et al., 1996; Stefanovic-Racic et al., 1994b, 1995
	Rat	Collagen-induced arthritis	Cannon et al., 1996
	Mouse	*Borrelia burgdorferi* (Lyme disease)	Seiler et al., 1995
	Mouse	MRL/*lpr* (lupus)	Weinberg et al., 1994

joints of patients with RA and osteoarthritis has confirmed the presence of iNOS mRNA and protein, and freshly isolated cartilage fragments continue to synthesize NO in culture. As discussed in Chapter 9, there is evidence that the cartilage of osteoarthritic joints expresses a dysregulated nNOS or a novel isoform of NOS known as 'OA-NOS' (Amin et al., 1995).

The data concerning NO production by human synovium are less uniform. It is possible to detect iNOS mRNA and protein in synovial tissues retrieved from arthritic, but not normal, joints (Sakurai et al., 1995), but it is not yet clear whether this tissue produces large amounts of NO. There is some disagreement as to which cells within the rheumatoid synovium express iNOS. The data of Sakurai and co-workers identified CD14[+] cells and endothelial cells as the major source of this enzyme (Sakuari et al., 1995). McInnes and co-workers, in contrast, identified synovial fibroblasts as the primary iNOS-containing cells (McInnes et al., 1996; see Chapters 2 and 5).

Synovial fluid leukocytes are another potential intra-articular source of NO, but Grabowski and co-workers were unable to detect its production by these cells (Grabowski et al., 1996b). Therefore, it remains possible that chondrocytes are the major intra-articular source of NO in human arthritis.

Despite considerable production of NO within diseased joints, it is likely that extra-articular tissues make important contributions to the NO derivatives detected in blood and urine. The findings of St Clair and co-workers suggest that blood monocytes could be one such source (St Clair et al., 1996). Data from studies with arthritic rats further identify the spleen, lymph and liver as important extra-articular sites of NO production in RA (Cannon et al., 1996).

In rodent models of arthritis, the increase in NO production usually precedes the onset of symptoms and it remains elevated during the chronic phase of the disease. These observations are consistent with the notion that NO may be involved in the initiation, as well as the progression, of rheumatoid disease. However, drug and

Table 6.3. *Effects of NOS inhibitors in experimental models of arthritis*

Model	Species	NOS inhibitor	Effect	Reference
Streptococcal cell wall	Rat	L-NAMA	Inhibition	McCartney-Francis et al., 1993
Adjuvant	Rat	L-NMA	Inhibition	Stefanovic-Racic et al., 1994b
		L-NAME	Inhibition	Ialenti et al., 1993
		Aminoguanidine	None	Stefanovic-Racic et al., 1995
		Aminoguanidine	Weak inhibition	Connor et al., 1995
		L-NIL	Inhibition	Connor et al., 1995
Collagen	Mouse	iNOS$^{-/-}$	None	Visco et al., 1997
K$_3$CrO$_8$	Mouse	DPI	Inhibition	Miesel et al., 1996
MRL/*lpr* (lupus)	Mouse	L-NMA	Inhibition	Weinberg et al., 1994
Borrelia burgdorferi (Lyme disease)	Mouse	L-NMA	None	Seiler et al., 1995

DPI, diphenylene iodonium chloride (inhibits NOS and other flavoproteins).

inhibitor studies, described below, caution against such simplistic assertions. Before reviewing the results of such studies, we will first consider what NO might be doing in arthritis.

6.3. Role of NO in arthritis pathophysiology

The major pathological lesions affecting arthritic joints are erosion of the cartilages and inflammation. Extra-articular manifestations of the disease can include weight loss, fever, arteritis and osteopenia. In RA, these changes are thought to be driven by autoimmune mechanisms. As these events can be viewed as dissociable pathophysiological processes, it is instructive to consider separately how NO might influence each of them.

The consequences of NO production for the integrity of articular cartilage are considered in Chapter 9 and will not be discussed again here. Suffice it to note that NO inhibits the synthesis of the major macromolecular components of cartilage; its effects on matrix breakdown remain to be determined to the satisfaction of all investigators.

Data concerning the role of NO in inflammation in general, and joint inflammation in particular, are confusing. The literature on these subjects is quite large and, in several places, contradictory. Depending upon how it is read, NO can be portrayed as an anti- or proinflammatory molecule (see Clancy and Abramson (1995), Evans (1995), Kubes and Wallace (1995), Miller and Grisham (1995) for reviews).

Studies on the role of NO in specific immunity are in their infancy and no clear picture is emerging. As with inflammation, the literature concerning NO and immunity contains inconsistencies, and instances can be found of immunosuppressive and immunostimulatory behaviour (Chapter 2; reviewed by Liew (1995) and Moilanen and Vapaatalo (1995)). Of interest is the possibility that NO could shift the balance between the activities of T_H1 and T_H2 lymphocytes. In mice, there is evidence that NO selectively suppresses T_H1 function (Taylor-Robinson *et al.*, 1994) and the iNOS 'knockout' mouse indeed exhibits a stronger T_H1 response than wild-type mice (Wei *et al.*, 1995). However, recent studies on human T lymphocytes failed to discern such selectively. Instead, NO was an inhibitor of both T_H1 and T_H2 activity (Bauer *et al.*, 1997).

From this brief account, it is clear that the effects of NOS inhibitors upon arthritis cannot be predicted from what is known of the properties of NO in related systems. With this in mind, the results of experiments in which NOS inhibitors have been introduced into animal models of arthritis will now be discussed.

6.4 Effects of NOS inhibitors in animal models of arthritis

The first models to be evaluated were adjuvant (Ialenti, Moncada and DiRosa, 1993; Stefanovic-Racic *et al.*, 1994b) and streptococcal cell wall (McCartney-Francis *et al.*, 1993) arthritis in rats (Table 6.3). Initial results were very promising. When administered prophylactically, L-NMA and L-NAME were able to suppress disease onset in a very dramatic fashion. Although these two inhibitors are not specific for iNOS, later work showed that L-NIL (*N*-iminoethyl-L-lysine), which inhibits iNOS to a much greater degree than it does cNOS, also possessed strong prophylactic activity in rat adjuvant arthritis (Connor *et al.*, 1995). Aminoguanidine, another NOS inhibitor with a certain degree of isoform specificity, was, however, without much effect (Connor *et al.*, 1995; Stefanovic-Racic *et al.*, 1995).

Disillusionment began with the observation that L-NMA, despite its strong prophylactic activity, has only weak therapeutic activity (Stefanovic-Racic *et al.*, 1995). Furthermore, murine collagen-induced arthritis was found to be resistant to NOS inhibitors as well as to disruption of the iNOS gene (Visco *et al.*, 1997). Studies in rats have shown that collagen induced arthritis provokes less NO synthesis than adjuvant arthritis (Cannon *et al.*, 1996). It was argued that strains of rats that are more susceptible to adjuvant arthritis excrete more urinary nitrate in response to adjuvant. Zidek and co-workers, however, could not confirm a similar relationship when studying NO production by peritoneal macrophages in this model (Zidek *et al.*, 1995).

Other evidence that the connection between NO production and disease severity may be imperfect comes from the use of anti-arthritic drugs. Indomethacin, for instance, has strong prophylactic and therapeutic activity in adjuvant arthritis in rats but has no consistent effect on the urinary excretion of nitrate (Stefanovic-Racic *et al.*, 1994b). Similarly, in human RA, treatment with prednisolone gives marked symptomatic improvement, with only modest reduction in urinary nitrate excretion (Stichtentoth *et al.*, 1995).

Prophylactic administration of NOS inhibitors has little effect on the extra-articular manifestations of RA (Table 6.4), except in the case of L-NAME, which protects against weight loss in adjuvant-induced arthritis, and aminoguanidine, which exacerbates weight loss in this model.

Table 6.4. *Effects of NOS inhibitors on extra-articular manifestations of disease in rat adjuvant arthritis*

Parameter	NOS inhibitor	Effect	Reference
Weight loss	L-NMA	None	Stefanovic-Racic *et al.*, 1994b
	L-NIL	None	Connor *et al.*, 1995
	L-NAME	Improved	Ialenti *et al.*, 1993
	Aminoguanidine	Exacerbated	Stefanovic-Racic *et al.*, 1995
Increased plasma fibrinogen	L-NMA	None	Stefanovic-Racic *et al.*, 1994b
	Aminoguanidine	None	Stefanovic-Racic *et al.*, 1995
Increased blood leukocyte count	L-NIL	None	Connor *et al.*, 1995

Unpublished information discussed informally among researchers in this area muddies the waters even further. It seems that, depending upon the animal model of choice, the NOS inhibitor employed and the route of administration of the inhibitor, disease may be prevented, exacerbated or unaffected. There are no published studies in which NOS inhibitors have been administered in animal models of osteoarthritis.

This all needs to be sorted out in a serious and careful manner. Part of the problem is the lack of an experimental model that satisfies all investigators as an authentic surrogate of human arthritis. This may mean that the only way to determine the role of NO in human arthritis will be to administer NOS inhibitors to patients. Such studies await the development of better isoform-specific inhibitors, as well as more advanced methods for measuring NO production *in vivo*. Human interventional trials will also need to be carefully designed to maximize the chance of detecting an effect on cartilage matrix metabolism; most protocols evaluate only the inflammatory component of the disease.

6.5 Conclusions

Despite convincing evidence that large amounts of NO are generated in RA, we still do not know whether NO is a mediator of disease, a protective agent or neither. Data obtained with animal models of disease are confusing and, if the unpublished findings discussed informally among investigators in this field pass muster, the published data are set to become even more confusing. The question is, where do we go from here? Several points should be made in this context.

As discussed earlier in this chapter, RA is a disease involving a number of interrrelated but distinct pathologies. It is quite possible that NO affects these different pathophysiological processes in different ways. NO could, for instance, prevent erosion of the articular cartilage while exacerbating the inflammatory response, or vice versa. It could also act differently in acute and chronic disease, and during flares its behaviour could be different again.

In terms of the possible clinical utility of NO agonists or antagonists, it is worth remembering that there already exist a number of anti-inflammatory drugs that, although not ideal, are reasonably useful agents for use in rheumatoid disease. To be clinically applied, novel anti-inflammatory drugs based upon NO would need to be more effective, cheaper or less prone to side-effects than existing drugs. Cartilage erosion is a different matter. It is not merely a secondary result of articular inflammation, and it is not arrested or reversed to any great degree by existing drugs. A chondroprotective drug based upon the modulation of NO would, there-fore, be of much greater significance. Moreover, it could find widespread use in the treatment of osteoarthritis where the major pathology is focal loss of articular cartilage. Before either of the above possibilities can be reduced to practice, there remains the need for much more basic research on the biology of both NO and arthritis.

Acknowledgements

The authors' work in this area has been supported by NIH grant AR42025. Lou Duerring typed the manuscript.

References

Amin, A. R., Cesare, P. E., Vyas, P. *et al.* (1995) The expression and regulation of nitric oxide synthase in human osteoarthritis-affected chondrocytes: evidence for up-regulated neuronal nitric oxide synthase. *J. Exp. Med.* **182**, 2097–2102.

Bauer, H., Jung, T., Tsikas, D., Stichtenoth, D. O., Frölich, J. C. and Neumann, C. (1997) Nitric oxide inhibits secretion of T-helper-1 and T-helper-2-associated cytokines in activated human T cells. *Immunology* **90**, 205–211.

Cannon, G. W., Openshaw, S. J., Hibbs, J. B., Hoidal, J. R., Huecksteadt, T. P and Griffiths, M. M. (1996) Nitric oxide production during adjuvant-induced and collagen-induced arthritis. *Arthritis Rheum.* **39**, 2677–2684.

Cao, M., Stefanovic-Racic, M., Greorgescu, H. I., Miller, L. A. and Evans, C. H. (1998) Generation of nitric oxide by lapine meniscal cells and its effects on collagen biosynthesis: stimulation of callogen production by arginine. *J. Orthop. Res.* in press.

Clancy, R. M. and Abramson, S. B. (1995) Nitric oxide: a novel mediator of inflammation. *Proc. Soc. Exp. Biol. Med.* **210**, 93–101.

Connor, J. R., Manning, P. T., Settle, S. L. *et al.* (1995) Suppression of adjuvant-induced arthritis by selective inhibition of inducible nitric oxide synthase. *Eur. J. Pharmacol.* **273**, 15–24.

Evans, C. H. (1995) Nitric oxide–what role does it play in inflammation and tissue destruction? In *Inflammation: Mechanisms and Therapeutics.* (ed. N. S. Doherty, B. M. Weichman, D. W. Morgan and L. Marshall). pp. 107–116. Birkhauser, Basel, Switzerland.

Evans, C. H. and Stefanovic-Racic, M. (1997) Nitric oxide in arthritis: it's probably there but what's it doing? In *Nitric Oxide, Cytochromes P450 and Sexual Steroid Hormones.* (ed. J. Lancaster and J. Parkinson). pp. 181–204. Springer-Verlag, Heidelberg.

Farrell, A. J., Blake, D. R., Palmer, R. M. and Moncada, S. (1992) Increased concentrations of nitrite in synovial fluid and serum suggest increased nitric oxide synthesis in rheumatic diseases. *Ann. Rheum. Dis.* **51**, 1219–1222.

Grabowski, P. S., England, A. J., Dykhuizen, R. *et al.* (1996a) Elevated nitric oxide production in rheumatoid arthritis: detection using the fasting urinary nitrate:creatinine ratio. *Arthritis Rheum.* **39**, 643–647.

Grabowski, P. S., Macpherson, H. and Ralston, S. M. (1996b) Nitric oxide production in cells derived from the human joint. *Br. J. Rheumatol.* **35**, 207–212.

Ialenti, A., Moncada, S. and DiRosa, M. (1993) Modulation of adjuvant arthritis by endogenous nitric oxide. *Br. J. Pharmacol.* **110**, 701–706.

Kaur, H. and Halliwell, B. (1994) Evidence for nitric oxide-mediated oxidative damage in chronic inflammation nitrotyrosine in serum and synovial fluid from rheumatoid patients. *FEBS Lett.* **350**, 9–12.

Kubes, P. and Wallace, J. L. (1995) Nitric oxide as a mediator of gastrointestinal mucosal injury? Say it ain't so. *Med. Inflam.* **4**, 397–405.

Liew, R. H. (1995) Regulation of lymphocyte functions by nitric oxide. *Curr. Opin. Immunol.* **7**, 396–399.

McCartney-Francis, N., Allen, J. B., Mizel, D. E. *et al.* (1993) Suppression of arthritis by an inhibitor of nitric oxide synthase. *J. Exp. Med.* **178**, 749–754.

McInnes, I. B., Leung, B. P., Field, M. *et al.* (1996) Production of nitric oxide in the synovial membrane of rheumatoid and osteoarthritis partients. *J. Exp. Med.* **184**, 1519–1524.

Miesel, R., Kurpisz, M. and Kroger, H. (1996) Suppression of inflammatory arthritis by simultaneous inhibition of nitric oxide synthase and NADPH oxidase. *Free Rad. Biol. Med.* **20**, 75–81.

Miller, M. J. S. and Grisham, M. B. (1995) Nitric oxide as a mediator of inflammation? You had better believe it. *Med. Inflam.* **4**, 387–396.

Moilanen, E. and Vapaatalo, H. (1995) Nitric oxide in inflammation and immune response. *Ann. Med.* **27**, 359–367.

Sakiniene, E., Bremell, T. and Tarkowski, A. (1996) Addition of corticosteroids to antibiotic treatment ameliorates the course of experimental *Staphlococcus aureus* arthritis. *Arthritis Rheum.* **39**, 1596–1605.

Sakurai, H., Kohsaka, H., Liu, M. F. *et al.* (1995) Nitric oxide production and inducible nitric oxide synthase expression in inflammatory arthritides. *J. Clin. Invest.* **96**, 2357–2363.

Seiler, K. P., Vavrin, Z., Eichwald, E., Hibbs, J. B. and Weiss, J. J. (1995) Nitric oxide production during murine Lyme disease: lack of involvement in host resistance or pathology. *Infect. Immun.* **63**, 3886–3895.

Stadler, J., Stefanovic-Racic, M., Billar, T. R. *et al.* (1991) Articular chondrocytes synthesize nitric oxide in response to cytokines and lipopolysaccharide. *J. Immunol.* **147**, 3915–3920.

St Clair, E. W., Wilkinson, W. E., Lang, T., Sanders, L., Misukonic, M. A. and Gilkinson, G. S. (1996) Increased expression of blood mononuclear cell nitric oxide synthase type 2 in rheumatoid arthritis patients. *J. Exp. Med.* **184**, 1173–1178.

Stefanovic-Racic, M. and Evans C. H. (1997) The role of nitric oxide in rheumatoid arthritis. In *Nitric Oxide Physiology and Pathophysiology.* (ed. G. Rubanyi). Birkhauser, Basel, in press.

Stefanovic-Racic, M., Stadler, J. and Evans, C. H. (1993) Nitric oxide and arthritis. *Arthritis Rheum.* **36**, 1036–1044.

Stefanovic-Racic, M., Stadler, J., Georgescu, H. I. and Evans, C. H. (1994a) Nitric oxide synthesis and its regulation by rabbit synoviocytes. *J. Rheumatol.* **21**, 1892–1898.

Stefanovic-Racic, M., Meyers, K., Meschter, C., Coffey, J. W., Hoffman, R. A. and Evans, C. H. (1994b) *N*-Monomethyl arginine, an inhibitor of nitric oxide synthase, suppresses the development of adjuvant arthritis in rats. *Arthritis Rheum.* **37**, 1062–1069.

Stefanovic-Racic, M., Meyers, K., Meschter, C., Coffey, J. W., Hoffman, R. A. and Evans, C. H. (1995) Comparison of the nitric oxide synthase inhibitors methylarginine and aminoguanidine as prophylactic and therapeutic agents in rat adjuvant arthritis. *J. Rheumatol.* **22**, 1922–1928.

Stichtentoth, D. O., Fauler, J., Zeidler, H. and Frölich, J. C. (1995) Urinary nitrate excretion is increased in patients with rheumatoid arthritis and reduced by prednisolone. *Ann. Rheum. Dis.* **54**, 820–824.

Taylor-Robinson, A. W., Liew, F. Y., Severn, A. *et al.* (1994) Regulation of the immune response by nitric oxide differentially produced by T helper type 1 and T helper type 2 cells. *Eur. J. Immounol.* **24**, 980–984.

Ueki, Y., Miyake, S., Tominaga, Y. and Eguchi, K. (1996) Increased nitric oxide levels in patients with rheumatiod arthritis. *J. Rheumatol.* **23**, 230–236.

Visco, D. M., Fletcher, D. S., Orevillo, C. J. *et al.* (1997) NOS 2 deficient mice are susceptible to collagen-induced arthritis. *Trans. Orthop. Res. Soc.* **22**, 416.

Wei, X. Q., Charles, I. G., Smith, A. *et al.* (1995) Altered immune responses in mice lacking inducible nitric oxide synthase. *Nature* **375**, 408–411.

Weinberg, J. B., Granger, D. L., Pisetsky, D. S. *et al.* (1994) The role of nitric oxide in the pathogenesis of spontaneous murine autoimmune disease: increased nitric production and nitric oxide synthase expression in MRL-*lpr*/*lpr* mice, and reduction of spontaneous glomerulonephritis and arthritis by orally adminstered N^{ω}-monomethyl-L-arginine. *J. Exp. Med.* **179**, 651–660.

Zidek, Z., Frankova, D. and Otava, B. (1995) Lack of causal relationship between inducibility/severity of adjuvant arthritis in the rat and disease associated changes in production of nitric oxide by macrophages. *Ann. Rheum. Dis.* **54**, 325–327.

7

Nitric oxide and prostaglandin interactions in acute and chronic inflammation

DANIELA SALVEMINI

7.1 Introduction

Substantial experimental evidence has been gathered over the years to demonstrate that NO plays important roles in acute and chronic inflammatory events. The distinct properties of each of the NOS isoforms have important implications since it is the magnitude, the duration and the cellular sites of NO production that determine the overall physiological or patho-physiological effect of NO. For example, release of NO from eNOS occurs in small amounts and for a short period of time. NO released under these circumstances plays a crucial role in the cardiovascular system where it controls organ blood flow distribution, inhibits the aggregation and adhesion of platelets to the vascular wall, inhibits leukocyte adhesion and inhibits smooth muscle cell proliferation (see Moncada and Higgs (1995) for review). In contrast, the inducible NOS isoform is not continuously present but is expressed in a variety of cells in response to inflammatory stimuli such as cytokines and LPS (Kroncke, Fehsel and Kolb-Bachofen, 1995). The net result is a delayed (typically 4–6 h) but very prolonged synthesis of high levels of NO. This sustained synthesis of NO derived from the action of iNOS has been implicated in acute and chronic inflammation as well as in host defence (Moncada and Higgs, 1995).

Besides the NOS system, COX, the enzyme that converts arachidonic acid to the prostaglandins, prostacyclin (PGI_2) and thromboxane A_2 (TXA_2) is another critical enzyme in many inflammatory diseases. Two forms of COX have been identified. The constitutive isoform (COX-1) is present in tissues such as the stomach, gut or kidney, where prostaglandin production plays a cytoprotective role in maintaining normal physiological processes (see Wu (1995) for review). In inflammatory processes, the inducible isoform COX-2 is expressed in many cells including fibroblasts and macrophages and accounts for the release of large quantities of proinflammatory prostaglandins at the site of inflammation (Wu, 1995).

An important property pertinent to the role of NO in inflammation is its ability to activate COX, resulting in substantial production of proinflammatory prostaglandins (Salvemini *et al.*, 1993). In this chapter, the multifaceted roles of NO and prostaglandins in inflammation are described, with a focus on the regulation of COX-2 activity by NO. COX-2 enzyme, once activated in the presence of NO, represents an important transduction mechanism for the actions of NO in acute and chronic inflammation.

7.2 NO, prostaglandins and inflammation

The potential for the production of sustained, high levels of NO from the iNOS as well as an increased understanding of the cytotoxic and/or cytostatic action of NO has led many investigators to examine the role of NO in a variety of patho-physiological conditions and is the subject of several recent reviews (Gross, 1995; Moilanen and Vapaatalo, 1995). Accumulating evidence indicates that excessive production of NO plays a pathogenic role in both acute and chronic models of inflammation (Clancy and Abramson, 1995; Moncada and Higgs, 1995). Two important discoveries have been made recently that may help to elucidate potential mechanisms of action of NO in inflammatory conditions. The first observation is that NO stimulates COX activity, resulting in the exaggerated production of proinflammatory prostaglandins (Salvemini *et al.* 1993). The second is that NO can react with O_2^- to form the cytotoxic radical peroxynitrite (Beckman *et al.*, 1990). NO is a potent vasodilator and its involvement during an inflammatory response may be related to its ability to increase vascular permeability and oedema through changes in local blood flow. NO is an important endogenous vasodilator of the human microcirculation, both in the rapid response to acetylcholine and in the delayed, steroid-sensitive response to an inflammatory stimulus (Warren, 1994). In an acute model of inflammation, Ialenti and co-workers (1992) and Salvemini and co-workers (1996a) demonstrated that two, non-selective NOS inhibitors, L-NAME and L-NMMA, attenuated the carrageenan- or dextran-induced oedema in the rat skin or paw. In acute inflammatory reactions in guinea-pig skin, Teixeira, Williams and Hellewell, (1993) demonstrated that L-NAME inhibited oedema formation and neutrophil accumulation. The authors speculate that the inhibitory action resulted from an inhibition of vasodilator tone in the microcirculation. Using more selective iNOS inhibitors such as L-NIL (Moore *et al.*, 1994; Connor *et al.*, 1995) to evaluate the roles of NO in this model, Salvemini and co-workers determined that NO synthesized from cNOS is responsible for the early development of inflammation in the carrageenan-induced rat paw model of inflammation whereas NO synthesized from iNOS is responsible for the later phase of the inflammatory response (Salvemini *et al.*, 1996a). Evidence also suggested that the mechanisms by which NO exerts its inflammatory response involves the release of prostaglandins (see below) and the formation of peroxynitrite (Salvemini *et al.*, 1996a).

Mulligan and co-workers (1991) used a rat model and L-NMMA to demonstrate that production of NO is linked to immune complex-induced tissue injury. Auto-reactive tissue destruction may also involve iNOS-derived NO production (Kolb and Kolb-Bachofen, 1992). A chronic, local inflammatory process occurs in the joints of patients with arthritis and the role of NO in the immune response, inflammation and tissue injury associated with arthritis has been recently reviewed (Stefanovic-Racic, Stadler and Evans, 1993). Increased concentrations of nitrite are observed in plasma and synovial fluid samples taken from patients with RA and osteoarthritis, suggesting an enhanced local synthesis of NO (Farrell *et al.*, 1992). In contrast, Kaur and Halliwell (1994) detected elevated levels of 3-nitrotyrosine (as a marker for peroxynitrite-dependent damage) in the blood serum and synovial fluid of patients with RA but not in patients with osteoarthritis. In a rat model of arthritis, induction of iNOS mRNA expression and elevated production of NO (measured as nitrite) was detected in synovial tissue and blood mononuclear cells (McCartney-Francis *et al.*, 1993). Furthermore, administration of L-NMMA reduced the accumulation of inflammatory leukocytes and reduced erosion of the joint. Urinary excretion of nitrite/nitrate (as an *in vivo* marker of NO production) was elevated in MRL *lpr/lpr* autoimmune mice and oral administration of L-NMMA attenuated both the spontaneous arthritis and glomerulonephritis (Weinberg *et al.*, 1994). The role of NO in arthritis has also been demonstrated by showing that L-NMMA (Stefanovic-Racic *et al.*, 1994) or L-NIL (Connor *et al.*, 1995) inhibited NO synthesis, paw swelling and histopathological changes in a rat model of adjuvant arthritis. Excessive release of NO from the inducible enzyme has also been implicated in hydronephrosis (Salvemini *et al.*, 1994), in the inflammatory response observed by the injection of carrageenan in the rat air pouch, where it plays an important role in neutrophil influx as well as in protein leakage (Salvemini *et al.*, 1995a), in sepsis and renal damage induced by endotoxin (Salvemini *et al.*, 1995b) and in glomerulonephritis (Cattell, Cook and Moncada, 1990; Cook and Sullivan, 1992). In these models, selective inhibitors of iNOS exert protective effects. The important role of NO in inflammation is that homozygous mutant mice lacking the iNOS gene show reduced inflammatory response to carrageenan when compared with the wild type or heterozygous mice (Wei, Charles and Smith, 1995).

Like NOS, COX has both constitutive and inducible isoforms. Synthesis of COX-2 is triggered by those cytokines that also induce iNOS and this may explain why iNOS and COX-2 are often expressed together in a variety of pathological states (Wu, 1995). There is now substantial evidence supporting the role of COX-2 as being primarily involved in both acute and chronic inflammation. Injection of carrageenan into a rat subcutaneous air pouch induces a rapid inflammatory response characterized by the induction of COX that coincides with the release of proinflammatory prostaglandins and thromboxane into the pouch exudate. Following carrageenan administration, COX-2 mRNA and protein is selectively induced in the rat air pouch and prostaglandins are significantly elevated in both the pouch lining and fluid exudate (Masferrer *et al.*, 1994a). The potent anti-inflammatory drug dexamethasone blocked the COX-2 induction and prostaglandin formation *in vivo*. Likewise, both non-selective NSAIDs (e.g. indomethacin) and selective COX-2 inhibitors (e.g. SC-58125, NS-398) blocked the prostaglandin release induced by carrageenan. However, in the same animals, indomethacin totally blocked stomach prostaglandin production while selective COX-2 inhibitors had no effect on gastric prostaglandin production. These results suggest that prostaglandin synthesis in the air pouch model is driven solely by COX-2 (Masferrer *et al.*, 1994a).

The rat carrageenan-induced paw model has been used traditionally to characterize NSAID anti-inflammatory and analgesic activity *in vivo*. Injection of carragee-nan into the hindpaw of the rat results in a rapid induction of oedema that is maximal at 3 h. This oedema corresponds to an abundant production of prostaglan-dins in the paw tissue, which is blocked by traditional NSAIDs. We correlated the formation of oedema to an induction of COX-2 mRNA in the paw, with no significant change in COX-1 expression (Seibert *et al.*, 1994). Likewise, selective inhibitors of COX-2 are anti-inflammatory in this model. In addition, selective COX-2 inhibitors inhibited carrageenan-induced hyperalgesia, consistent with a clinical requirement that an NSAID relieve inflammatory pain (Seibert *et al.*, 1994).

Both Dup697 and NS-398 (selective COX-2 inhibitor) have been reported to inhibit the inflammatory response in an adjuvant-induced model of arthritis (Gans *et al.*, 1989; Futaki *et al.*, 1993a,b). We evaluated the role of COX-2 in this arthritis model and observed an induction of COX-2 mRNA and protein that correlated with the induction of prostaglandin production in the inflamed joint and the incidence of oedema. Therapeutic administration of selective inhibitors of COX-2 blocked the production of prostaglandins as well as the oedema in these chronically inflamed animals (Masferrer *et al.*, 1994b).

In summary, it is clear that the iNOS and COX-2 systems are often present together, share a number of similarities and play fundamental roles in acute and chronic inflammation . An additional feature that links the NOS and COX pathways in inflammation is that NO can markedly enhance the production of proinflamma-tory prostaglandins, resulting in an exacerbation and continuation of the inflamma-tory response (Salvemini *et al.*, 1993). This property of NO is attributable to its ability to activate the COX enzymes (Salvemini *et al.*, 1993). This discovery was made initially in *in vitro* systems and subsequently in *in vivo* studies. Its importance in inflammation was then evaluated in various models of acute and chronic inflammatory conditions.

7.3 Activation of COX-2 by NO: discovery

iNOS and COX-2 enzymes can be induced in macrophages following stimulation with endotoxin; this results in a large production of NO and prostaglandins. Inhibition of iNOS activity by non-selective NOS inhibitors, such as L-NMMA or L-NNA, or more selective iNOS inhibitors, such as L-NIL or aminoguanidine (Corbett *et al.*, 1992; Misko *et al.*, 1993; Moore *et al.*, 1994; Connor *et al.*, 1995), attenuate the large production of NO from these cells. As NO release was inhibited so was the release of the prostaglandins (Salvemini *et al.*, 1993). The NOS inhibitors did not behave as NSAIDs for they did not inhibit COX activity (Salvemini *et al.*, 1993); nor did they affect the induction of COX-2 (unpublished observations). These results suggested that endogenously released NO from the macrophages exerted a stimulatory action on COX-2 activity, enhancing the production of prostaglandin. Therefore, inhibition of NOS activity reduced the output of prostaglandins from COX-2.

To further support a direct role of NO on COX-2 activity, IL-1β-stimulated human fibroblast cells (which do not possess an endogenous L-arginine to NO pathway) were tested in the presence of exogenous NO. Exposure of IL-1β-stimulated fibroblasts to either NO gas or two NO donors (sodium nitroprusside and glyceryl trinitrate) increased COX activity by at least fourfold; this resulted in increased production of prostaglandin. This phenomenon is independent of the known effects of NO on the soluble guanylyl cyclase. Methylene blue, an inhibitor of the soluble guanylyl cyclase, inhibited the increase in cGMP by NO in the fibroblast but did not prevent its ability to stimulate COX activity and hence prostaglandin production (Salvemini *et al.*, 1993).

The most likely explanation for the mechanism by which NO activates COX is a direct stimulation of the enzyme. Indeed we demonstrated that NO could directly increase COX activity of microsomal sheep seminal vesicles (Salvemini *et al.*, 1995c) as well as murine recombinant COX-1 and COX-2 (Salvemini *et al.*, 1993). Although the molecular mechanism by which NO activates COX remains to be identified, a few possibilities exist. NO interacts with oxygen-derived free radicals such as superoxide anions (Gryglewski, Palmer and Moncada, 1989). Interaction between NO and O_2^- leads to the formation of peroxynitrite, which can then decompose to form the hydroxyl radical (Beckman *et al.*, 1990). Therefore, NO may augment COX activity by acting as an anti-oxidant (removal of O_2^-) or by generating $ONOO^-$ and OH', which subsequently activate COX. Indeed, it is known that free radicals such as O_2^- and OH' modulate the COX pathway (Egan, Paxton and Kuehl, 1976). In addition, it has been recently reported that NO nitrosylates cysteine residues in the catalytic domain of COX enzymes, leading to its activation (Hajjar *et al.*, 1995).

7.4 Activation of COX-2 by NO: implications in acute and chronic inflammation

In vivo studies revealed that the regulation of COX by NO is a powerful mechanism that is used by NO to amplify the course of the inflammatory response. Indeed, we and others observed that iNOS and COX-2 are induced in a number of inflammatory models, including rabbit hydronephrotic kidney (Salvemini *et al.*, 1994), endotoxin-induced septic shock (Salvemini *et al.*, 1995b) and carrageenan-induced pouch and paw inflammation (Vane *et al.*, 1994; Salvemini *et al.*, 1995a, 1996a; Swierkosz *et al.*, 1995). The prolonged release of large amounts of NO and prostaglandin may subsequently lead to deleterious effects. Inhibition of NO release by selective iNOS inhibitors is associated with profound inhibition of prostaglandin release; the anti-inflammatory potency of the iNOS inhibitors correlated with their respective ability to block both NO and prostaglandin release (Vane *et al.*, 1994; Salvemini *et al.*, 1995a, 1996a; Swierkosz *et al.*, 1995). For instance, in an acute model of inflammation (carrageenan-induced paw oedema in rats), inhibition of oedema with L-NIL is associated with a dose-dependent inhibition of NO release and a clear inhibition of proinflammatory prostaglandin release (Salvemini *et al.*,

1996a); inhibition of NO production in lungs taken from endotoxin-treated rats has also been shown to result in an inhibition of prostacyclin release (Sautebin and Di Rosa, 1994).

Injection of carrageenan into the pre-formed air pouch of a rat induces an inflammatory response characterized by iNOS and COX-2 induction, white blood cell infiltration, oedema and protein leakage into the pouch (Salvemini *et al.*, 1995a). Selective inhibition of iNOS by L-NIL and aminoguanidine inhibited not only NO production but also prostaglandin production (Salvemini *et al.*, 1995a). All other parameters of inflammation were attenuated; histological examination of the pouch lining taken from animals treated with the iNOS inhibitor revealed a lack of inflammation (Salvemini *et al.*, 1995a). In this scenario, we were able to demonstrate that in the presence of L-NIL, COX-2 was activated at least sevenfold by exogenous injection of NO donors such as sodium nitroprusside or nitroglycerin; this activation resulted in a profound increase in PGE_2 release (Salvemini *et al.*, 1995a). Similar results have been observed in the hydronephrotic rabbit model of inflammation (Salvemini *et al.*, 1994). That the proinflammatory roles of NO have a prostaglandin component has also been demonstrated by showing that the injection of sodium nitroprusside elicits oedema in the footpad of rats and the formation of this oedema is blocked by NSAIDs (Sautebin *et al.*, 1995). Therefore, the effects of endogenously released NO on COX-2 are mimicked by exogenous NO. Regulation of COX-2 by iNOS-derived NO is a powerful mechanism that amplifies the course of the inflammatory response. In this respect, the dual inhibition of proinflammatory NO and prostaglandin production contributes to the anti-inflammatory properties of the NOS inhibitors observed in a number of models.

Although for the purpose of this chapter, it was not discussed in any great detail, it is important to remember that the interactions between these pathways is not limited to the inflammatory response. Indeed we and others have demonstrated that NO derived from the constitutive form of the NOS enzyme activates COX-1, and this has important consequences in normal physiological conditions (see Salvemini *et al.*, (1996b) for review). In addition, the discovery that NO activates COX-1 to release cytoprotective prostaglandins raises the possibility that the increased platelet aggregation, vasoconstriction and elevation of systemic blood pressure induced by inhibition of endogenous NO production by non-selective NOS inhibitors could be caused not only by removal of endogenous NO but also by a concurrent reduction of anti-platelet and vasodilator COX products. Dual inhibition of NO and prostaglandin production by non-selective NOS inhibitors may well explain the deleterious effects observed with these drugs in organs such as the kidneys and gastrointestinal tract, where both NO and prostaglandins exert cytoprotection.

7.5 Perspectives of NO-driven COX interactions in inflammation

The production of low amounts of NO and prostaglandins from the constitutive enzymes appears to regulate a number of important physiological processes, including the inhibition of platelet aggregation and white blood cell adhesion, regulation of blood vessel tone and cytoprotection in the kidney and intestinal mucosa. Non-selective inhibitors of NOS are capable of causing damage to the gut and kidney, a property shared by NSAIDs. It is possible that the deleterious effect of the non-selective NOS inhibitors results from blockade of not only NO production but also of prostaglandin production (released as a consequence of NO-mediated COX-1 activation). It is, therefore, imperative to preserve cNOS and COX-1 activity in an inflammatory setting; this can be achieved by the use of glucocorticoids. The potent anti-inflammatory glucocorticoid dexamethasone is a good example of dual iNOS (Moncada and Higgs, 1995) and COX-2 (Masferrer and Seibert, 1994) inhibition. Unfortunately, serious side-effects of steroids, independent of their ability to block iNOS and COX-2 expression, limit their clinical usage. Selective inhibition of iNOS or COX-2 is also anti-inflammatory in a number of models. Besides its proinflammatory role, a feature of NO that is not shared by prostaglandins is its potent cytotoxic effect. This could explain why in arthritis a NSAID such as indomethacin, by blocking prostaglandin but not NO production, alleviates the symptoms associated with the inflammatory insult but does not modify the course of the disease (Flynn, 1994). Since selective iNOS inhibitors have the potential of reducing both NO and prostaglandin, it is exciting to consider that the utilization of these selective iNOS inhibitors may have the advantage of not only alleviating inflammatory symptoms through dual inhibition of NO and NO-driven COX-2 activation but also of eliminating further cytotoxic damage of NO, these may prove to be important disease-modifying drugs in chronic inflammatory diseases such as RA. Amplification of the inflammatory response by NO-driven COX-2 activation is depicted in Figure 7.1.

7.6 Conclusions

This chapter highlights the importance, in the context of inflammation, of the discovery that COX enzymes are activated by NO. We have demonstrated that in inflammatory conditions in which the iNOS and COX-2 systems are induced there is an NO-mediated increase in the production of large quantities of proinflammatory prostaglandins; this results in an exacerbated inflammatory response. Since our initial findings on the regulation of COX enzymes by NO, there is now a growing body of experimental evidence emerging from the literature that supports the importance of the NO-mediated COX activation in the regulation and amplification of physio-pathological events (e.g. Corbett *et al.*, 1993; Davidge *et al.*, 1995; Inoue *et al.*, 1993; Mollace *et al.*, 1995). Further understanding of how these two critical systems interact will undoubtedly provide us with a novel way to tackle acute and chronic inflammatory events. Although not discussed in any great detail or length, it is also evident that the activation of COX-1 by NO may represent an important mechanism through which NO and prostaglandins can exert their beneficial cytoprotective effects in the cardiovascular system and in the

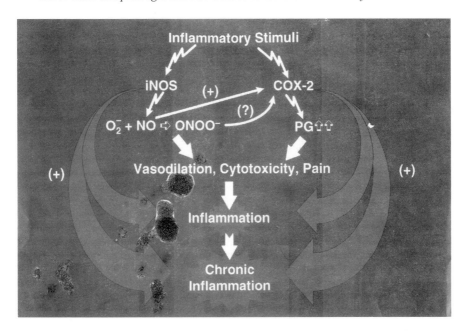

Figure 7.1. Amplification of the inflammatory response following NO-driven COX-2 activation. Mediators released during the course of an inflammatory stimulus (e.g. cytokines) induce iNOS and COX-2, which in turn release large amounts of proinflammatory NO and prostaglandins. Free radicals such as superoxide anions (O_2^-) are also produced by neutrophils that infiltrate into the inflamed site. These mediators alone or through synergistic interactions with other mediators initiate a series of events that are associated with the inflammatory response (e.g. vasodilatation, cytotoxicity, pain). After a while, the inflammatory response wanes off (acute). In some instances, NO through continuous activation of COX-2 allows for more and more proinflammatory prostaglandins to be generated, setting in motion a vicious circle that allows the inflammatory response to continue. This could perhaps be one of the mechanisms that allows acute inflammatory response to evolve into a more chronic one. Although not known, it is also possible that peroxynitrite ($ONOO^-$) contributes to COX-2 activation (see review).

central nervous system. Furthermore, the activation of COX-1 by NO is an alternative mechanism by which clinically used NO donors can exert their therapeutic effects (Salvemini *et al.*, 1996c). The NO-driven COX-1 activation also seems to have a role in reproduction in that NO stimulates the secretion of luteinizing hormone-releasing hormone from the hypothalamus (Rettori *et al.*, 1992) and modulates uterine motility (Franchi *et al.*, 1994) by activating COX-1 and releasing PGE_2. These are all exciting areas that need to be explored in the future.

The soluble guanylyl cyclase has been considered for many years to be the sole endogenous receptor for the actions of NO. This can no longer be the case. In fact, the broader implication of our discovery that NO activates COX is that the COX enzymes are also endogenous 'receptors' for the physiological and pathological effects of NO.

References

Beckman, J. S., Beckman, T. W., Chen, T. W., Marshall, P. A. and Freeman, B. A. (1990) Apparent hydroxyl radical production by peroxynitrite: implications for endothelial injury from nitric oxide and superoxide. *Proc. Natl. Acad. Sci., USA* **87**, 1620–1624.

Cattell, V., Cook, T. and Moncada, S. (1990) Glomeruli synthesize nitrite in experimental nephrotoxic nephritis. *Kidney Int.* **38**, 1056–1060.

Clancy, R. M. and Abramson, S. B. (1995) Nitric oxide: a novel mediator of inflammation. *Soc. Exp. Biol. Med.* **23**, 93–101.

Connor, J., Manning, P. T., Settle, S. L. *et al.* (1995) Suppression of adjuvant-induced arthritis by selective inhibition of inducible nitric oxide synthase. *Eur. J. Pharmacol.* **273**, 15–24.

Cook, H. Y. and Sullivan, R. (1992) Glomerular nitrate synthesis *in situ* in immune complex glomerulonephritis in the rat. *Am. J. Phatol.* **139**, 1047–1052.

Corbett, J. A., Tilton, R. G., Chang, K. *et al.*, (1992) Aminoguanidine, a novel inhibitor of nitric oxide formation, prevents diabetic vascular dysfunction. *Diabetes* **41**, 552–556.

Corbett, J. A., Kwon, G., Turk, J. and McDaniel, M. L. (1993) IL1β induces the coexpression of both nitric oxide synthase and cyclooxygenase by islets of Langerhans: activation of cyclooxygenase by nitric oxide. *Biochemistry* **32**, 13 767–13 770.

Davidge, S. T., Baker, P. N., Mclaughlin, M. K. and Roberts, J. M. (1995) Nitric oxide produced by endothelial cells increases production of eicosanoids through activation of prostaglandin H synthase. *Circ. Res.* **77**, 274–283.

Egan, R. W., Paxton, J. and Kuehl, F. A. Jr (1976) Mechanism for irreversible self-deactivation of prostaglandin synthetase. *J. Biol. Chem.* **251**, 7329–7335.

Farrell, A. J., Blake, D. R., Palmer, R. M. and Moncada, S. (1992) Increased concentrations of nitrite in synovial fluid and serum samples suggest increased nitric oxide synthesis in rheumatic diseases, *Ann. Rheum. Dis.* **51**, 1219–1222.

Flynn, B. L. (1994) Rheumatoid arthritis and osteoarthritis: current and future therapies. *Am. Pharm.* **NS34**, 31–42.

Franchi, A. M., Chaud, M., Rettori, V., Suburu, A., McCann, S. M. and Gimeno, M. (1994) Role of nitric oxide in eicosanoid synthesis and uterine motility in estrogen-treated rat uteri. *Proc Natl. Acad. Sci., USA.* **91**, 539–543.

Futaki, N., Yoshikawa, K., Yumiko, H. *et al.* (1993a) NS-398, a novel non-steroidal anti-inflammatory drug with potent analgesic and antipyretic effects which cause minimal stomach lesions. *Gen. Pharmacol.* **24**, 105–110.

Futaki, N., Arai, I., Hamasaki, S., Takahashi, S., Higuchi, S. and Otomo, S. (1993b) Selective inhibition of NS-398 on prostanoid production in inflammatory tissues in rat carrageenan-air-pouch inflammation. *J. Pharm. Pharmacol.* **45**, 753–755.

Gans, K. R., Galbraith, W., Roman, R. J. *et al.* (1989) Anti-inflammatory and safety profile of DuP 697, a novel orally effective prostaglandin synthesis inhibitor. *J. Pharm. Exp. Ther.* **254**, 180–185.

Gross, S. S. (1995) Nitric oxide: pathophysiological mechanisms *Annu. Rev. Physiol.* **57**, 737–769.

Gryglewski, R. J., Palmer, R. M. J. and Moncada, S. (1987) Superoxide anion is involved in the breakdown of endothelium-derived vascular relaxing factor. *Nature,* **320**, 454–456.

Hajjar, D. P., Lander, H. M., Pearce, F. S., Upmacis, R. K and Pomerantz, K. B. (1995) Nitric oxide enhances prostaglandin-H synthase activity by a heme-independent mechanism: evidence implicating nitrosothiols. *J. Am. Chem. Soc.* **117**, 3340–3346.

Ialenti, A., Ianaro, A., Moncada, S. and Di Rosa, M. (1992) Modulation of acute inflammation by endogenous nitric oxide. *Eur. J. Pharmacol* **211**, 177–182.

Inoue, T., Fukuo, K., Morimoto, S., Koh, E. and Ogihara, T. (1993) Nitric oxide mediates interleukin-1-induced prostaglandin E_2 production by vascular smooth muscle cells. *Biochem. Biophys. Res. Commun.* **194**, 420–424.

Kaur, H. and Halliwell, B. (1994) Evidence for nitric oxide-mediated oxidative damage in chronic inflammation. *FEBS Lett.* **350**, 9–12.

Kolb, H. and Kolb-Bachofen, V. (1992) Nitric oxide: a pathogenic factor in autoimmunity. *Immunol. Today* **13**, 157–159.

Kroncke, K.-D., Fehsel, K. and Kolb-Bachofen, V. (1995) Inducible nitric oxide synthase and its product nitric oxide, a small molecule with complex biological activities. *Biol. Chem.* **376**, 327–343.

Masferrer, J. L. and Seibert, K. (1994) Regulation of prostaglandin synthesis by glucocorticoids. *Receptor* **94**, 25–30.

Masferrer, J. L., Zweifel, B. S., Manning, P. T. *et al.* (1994a) Selective inhibition of inducible cyclooxygenase 2 *in vivo* is antiinflammatory and nonulcerogenic. *Proc. Natl. Acad. Sci., USA* **91**, 3228–3232.

Masferrer, J., Reddy, S., Zweifel, B. *et al.* (1994b) *In vivo* regulation of cyclooxygenase-2 by glucocorticoids in peritoneal macrophages. *J. Pharm. Exp. Ther.* **270**, 1340–1345.

McCartney-Francis, N., Allen, J. B., Mizel, D. E. *et al.* (1993) Suppression of arthritis by an inhibitor of nitric oxide synthase. *J. Exp. Med.* **178**, 749–754.

Misko, T. P., Moore, W. M., Kasten, T. P. *et al.* (1993) Selective inhibition of the inducible nitric oxide synthase by aminoguanidine. *Eur. J. Pharmacol.* **233**, 119–125.

Moilanen, E. and Vapaatalo, H. (1995) Nitric oxide in inflammation and immune response. *Ann. Med.* **27**, 359–367.

Mollace, V., Colasanti, V., Rodino, P., Lauro, G. M., Rotiroti, D. and Nistico, G. (1995) NMDA-dependent prostaglandin E_2 release by human cultured astroglial cells is driven by nitric oxide. *Biochem. Biophys. Res. Commun.* **215**, 793–799.

Moncada, S. and Higgs, E. A. (1995) Molecular mechanisms and therapeutic strategies related to nitric oxide. *FASEB J.* **9**, 1319–1330.

Moore, W. M., Webber, R. K., Jerome, G. M., Tjoeng, F. S., Misko, T. P. and Currie, M. G. (1994) L-N6-(1-iminoethyl)lysine: a selective inhibitor of inducible nitric oxide synthase. *J. Med. Chem.* **37**, 3886–3888.

Mulligan, M. S., Hevel, J. M., Marletta, M. A. and Ward, P. A. (1991) Tissue injury caused by deposition of immune complexes is L-arginine dependent. *Proc. Nat. Acad. Sci., USA* **88**, 6338–6342.

Rettori, V., Gimeno, M., Lyson, K. and McCann, S. M. (1992) Nitric oxide mediates norepinephrine-induced prostaglandin E_2 release from the hypothalamus. *Proc. Nat. Acad. Sci., USA* **89**, 11 543–11 546.

Salvemini, D., Misko, T. P., Masferrer, J. L., Seibert, K., Currie, M. G. and Needleman, P. (1993) Nitric oxide activates cyclooxygenase enzymes. *Proc. Natl. Acad. Sci. USA* **90**, 7240–7244.

Salvemini, D., Seibert, K., Masferrer, J. L., Misko, T. P., Currie, M. G. and Needleman, P. (1994) Endogenous nitric oxide enhances prostaglandin production in a model of renal inflammation. *J. Clin. Invest.* **93**, 1940–1947.

Salvemini, D., Manning, P. T., Zweifel, B. S. *et al.* (1995a) Dual inhibition of nitric oxide and prostaglandin production contributes to the antiinflammatory properties of nitric oxide synthase inhibitors. *J. Clin. Invest.* **96**, 301–308.

Salvemini, D., Settle, S. L., Masferrer, J. L., Seibert, K., Currie, M. G. and Needleman, P. (1995b) Regulation of prostaglandin production by nitric oxide: an *in vivo* analysis. *Br. J. Pharmacol.* **114**, 1171–1178.

Salvemini, D., Misko, T. P., Masferrer, J., Seibert, K., Currie, M. G. and Needleman, P. (1995c) In *Biology of Nitric Oxide*, 4: *Enzymology, Biochemistry and Immunology*. (ed. S. Moncada, M. Feelish and R. Busse) Portland Press, London.

Salvemini, D., Wang, Z. Q., Wyatt, P. S. *et al.* (1996a) Nitric oxide: a key mediator in the early and late phase of carrageenan-induced rat paw inflammation. *Br. J. Pharmacol.* **118**, 829–838.

Salvemini, D., Seibert, K. and Marino, M. H. (1996b) Prostaglandin release, as a consequence of NO-driven COX activation, contributes to the proinflammatory effects of NO: new concepts in inflammation and therapy. *DN&P*, **9**, 204–215.

Salvemini, D., Currie, M. G. and Mollace, V. (1996c) Nitric oxide-mediated cyclooxygenase activation: a key event in the antiplatelet effects of nitrovasodilators. *J. Clin. Invest.* **97**, 2562–2568.

Sautebin, L. and Di Rosa, M. (1994) Nitric oxide modulates prostacyclin biosynthesis in the lung of endotoxin-treated rats. *Eur. J. Pharmacol.* **262**, 193–196.

Sautebin, L., Ialenti, A., Ianaro, A. and Di Rosa, M. (1995) Modulation by nitric oxide of prostaglandin biosynthesis in the rat. *Br. J. Pharmacol.* **114**, 323–328.

Seibert, K., Zhang, Y., Leahy, K. *et al.* (1994) Pharmacological and biochemical demonstration of the role of cyclooxygenase 2 in inflammation and pain, *Proc. Natl. Acad. Sci., USA* **91**, 12 013–12 017.

Stefanovic-Racic, M., Stadler, J. and Evans, C. H. (1993) Nitric oxide and arthritis. *Arthritis Rheum.* **36**, 1036–1044.

Stefanovic-Racic, M., Meyers, K., Meschter, C., Coffey, J. W., Hoffman, R. A. and Evans, C. H. (1994) *N*-Monomethyl arginine, an inhibitor of nitric oxide synthase, suppresses the development of adjuvant arthritis in rats. *Arthritis Rheum.* **7**, 1062–1069.

Swierkosz, T. A., Mitchell, J. A. Warner, T. D., Botting, R. M. and Vane, R. (1995) Co-induction of nitric oxide synthase and cyclooxygenase: interactions between nitric oxide and prostanoids. *Br. J. Pharmacol.* **114**, 1335–1342.

Teixeira, M. M., Williams, T. J. and Hellewell, P. G. (1993) Role of prostaglandins and nitric oxide in acute inflammatory reactions in guinea-pig skin. *Br. J. Pharmacol.* **110**, 1515–1521.

Vane, J. R., Mitchell, J. A., Appleton, I. *et al.* (1994) Inducible isoforms of cyclooxygenase and nitric-oxide synthase in inflammation. *Proc. Natl. Acad. Sci., USA* **91**, 2046–2050.

Warren, J. B. (1994) Nitric oxide and human skin blood flow responses to acetylcholine and ultraviolet light, *FASEB J.* **8**, 247–251.

Wei, X., Charles, I. G. and Smith, A. (1995) Altered immune responses in mice lacking inducible nitric oxide synthase. *Nature* **375**, 408–412.

Weinberg, J. B., Granger, D. L., Pisetsky, D. S. *et al* (1994) The role of nitric oxide in the pathogenesis of spontaneous murine autoimmune disease: increased nitric oxide production and nitric oxide synthase expression in MRL-*lpr/lpr* mice, and reduction of spontaneous glomerulonephritis and arthritis by orally administered N^{ω}-monomethyl-L-arginine. *J. Exp. Med.* **179**, 651–660.

Wu, K. K. (1995) Inducible cyclooxygenase and nitric oxide synthase. *Adv. Pharmacol.* **33**, 179–207.

8

The complex influences of reactive oxygen species on rheumatoid erosions and synovitis

JANOS M. KANCZLER, TULIN SAHINOGLU, CLIFF R. STEVENS and DAVID R. BLAKE

8.1 Introduction

Rheumatoid arthritis (RA) may be defined, in part, as an example of an often persistent symmetrical synovitis that is associated with erosive bone and cartilage damage, both of which contribute to a progressive loss of joint function. Although there are a number of persistent inflammatory forms of synovitis that are not associated with erosive bone damage, there are other conditions such as psoriatic arthritis and crystal-induced arthritis where erosive damage is a feature but the location and nature of the damage are distinctive and different from that in RA. Conversely, in inflammatory forms of osteoarthritis, erosions are not a feature. Indeed an osteophytic, perhaps reparative, stabilizing response is a hallmark of the pathology. In inflammatory mediators cause bone erosion then clearly their influence on the process is complex.

8.2 Where do erosions develop?

In infective arthritis, where the relationship between synovial inflammation and erosive bone damage appears to be the most direct, erosions are found in the bare areas where the synovium directly abuts the bone. In chronic granulomatous states, the absence of significant loss of joint space in the presence of juxta-articular osteopenia and erosions characterize the damage. In RA, a periarticular osteopenia is an early feature of disease, thought to occur as a result of changes to synovial blood flow. In addition, three different forms of erosive damage are found as well as subchondral cyst formation (reviewed in Resnick, Bernthiaume and Sartoris, 1993). The first is the marginal erosion that occurs at bare sites. Such sites are also in close physical proximity to the insertion of the capsule ligaments, an area that is believed to be considerably innervated. Compressive erosions develop when osteopenic bones collapse or one bone invaginates another. In the third type of erosion, surface erosions, bone underlying inflamed tendons is resorbed. This process most characteristically occurs around the ulnar styloid process in the wrist. These broad clinical descriptions favour the conclusion that inflammation in the overlying tissue, either synovium or tendon sheath, is the major driving force for the initial erosive pathology. The possibility must also be considered that microerosions breaking the periosteal surface release bone debris that may initiate synovial inflammation and augment the damage.

8.3 Erosions, symmetry and the nervous system

Erosions often have strikingly symmetrical distribution, particularly in early rheumatoid disease. Asymmetry of erosion development may occur if RA follows an upper motor neurone hemiplegia or poliomyelitis. Both erosion and synovitis are attenuated on the affected side, suggesting that neurogenic factors influence the symmetry of the erosive process (Kidd, Cruwys and Polak, 1990). This process is complex, as denervation in the absence of an inflammatory synovitis (Charcot's neuropathic arthropathy) is associated with both a hypotrophic response, with new bone formation, and an atrophic pattern, with resorption of fragmented osteocarti-lage debris. How much of these changes relate to neuropeptide release or neuropep-tide loss and how much to the effects of trauma or joint laxity remain very unclear. The complex effects of neuropeptides, such as substance P or CGRP, on the vascular system via the release of NO, however, may explain some forms of acro-osteolysis related to a developing diabetic neuropathy, which is associated with neuropeptide release from progressively ischaemic peripheral nerves.

8.4 Movement and erosions

A form of erosive rheumatoid disease referred to as 'typus robustus arthritis' occurs for the most part in men who typically use their joints excessively. Large erosions and subchondral cysts, which may fracture, are a characteristic feature and suggest an influence of movement on the erosive process. Figure 8.1 is a radiograph of a right-handed professional jazz drummer, who succeeded in working despite devel-oping RA. It demonstrates very severe erosive damage. The asymmetric nature of the pathology highlights the probable influence of movement on joint pathology (see caption). In contrast, fusion of joints, which occurs following a fixed flexion deformity, appears to halt erosive development. Movement may of course explain in part some of the asymmetrical erosive disease found following a hemiplegia that precedes the development of RA. The influence of movement on the 'redox' state of the joint is discussed below.

8.5 Erosions and therapy

Our ability to suppress erosions in RA remains a much debated topic, but, at best, present therapies have a minimal anti-erosive effect. Steroids may suppress erosive development in the short term but the effects are not dramatic and are thought to be independent of an effect on synovitis (Kirwan, 1995). For other disease-modifying agents such as gold, penicillamine and methotrexate, the anti-erosive effects, when treatment is started late, are very poor. Treatment with second-line drugs is now

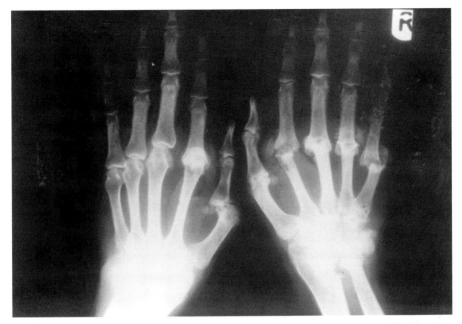

Figure 8.1 Male patient with RA showing gross erosive damage of wrist, small joints of the hand and select metacarpal joints. He was employed as a jazz drummer manipulating his drumsticks across his right hand but holding the stick only across the first three fingers of the left. Note the asymmetrical distribution of the affected joints.

advocated early following the onset of disease. Despite much rhetoric, there are, however, still no data to suggest that early aggressive therapy will halt erosion development. Despite the fact that there is a clear effect on synovitis of non-steroidal COX inhibitors, it is evident that such drugs neither halt erosions nor suppress their development. Given the apparent relationship of synovitis and erosions, and the ability of these compounds partially to suppress synovitis, our failure to show any effect on the erosive process requires an explanation. Is it because one requires the effect of the anti-inflammatory compound to be much more dramatic? In which case steroids should have a very demonstrable effect. Or is it because there is something about the pathological basis of synovitis that is not influenced by these drugs. We argue below that hypoxia is a major force in transforming cells within the synovium to a locally invasive phenotype. Our present therapies do not significantly influence the biochemical process specific to hypoxic injury and driven by hypoxia-specific transcription factors through hypoxia-response elements controlling gene transcription.

In order to understand the complexity and subtlety of the erosive process, we now review the multiple mediator systems generated within the synovium and established as having an influence on osteoblast–osteoclast coupling. We will then examine the nature of the joint environment, which alters the cellular and extracellular redox balance and modulates cytokine effects, and relate this to the clinical observations above. Finally, we will consider the influence of redox disturbances on a specific oxidoreductase, xanthine oxidase, which we hypothesize plays a critical role in maintaining synovial inflammation, and on both coupling and uncoupling osteoblast–osteoclast responses.

8.6 A question of balance

To maintain skeletal integrity, bone is constantly remodelling. This requires the amount of bone resorption to balance the amount of bone formation. When this process is imbalanced towards resorption, as in the case of RA or osteoporosis, bone loss is inevitable. Since the 1970s, considerable advances have been made in our understanding of the basic cellular mechanisms that regulate the formation and activity of the osteoclast. Though the osteoclast is the pivotal resorptive cell, the osteoblast is crucial in influencing the resorptive process. The bone microenvironment involves a complex sequence of cellular events occurring at specific regions. Site-specific signals that can promote cell differentiation, proliferation and coupling must occur at the correct time in the sequence of bone remodelling. With so many factors implicated in regulating this mechanism, it is understandable that a slight variation in this complex may result in a chaotically driven pathology.

8.7 Multiple mediators of bone resorption: a recipe for chaos?

Table 8.1 lists the vast array of agents that can influence bone resorption under physiological and pathological conditions. The main influences appear to be the systemic hormones, cytokines, growth factors and, identified more recently, reactive oxygen and nitrogen species (reviewed in Bilezikian, Raisz and Rodan, 1996).

8.7.1 Hormonal modulation

The systemic hormones PTH and 1,25-dihdroxy vitamin D_3 influence osteoclastic bone resorption. PTH is a central component of calcium homeostasis through its actions to reclaim filtered calcium in the kidney, to facilitate absorption of calcium from the gastrointestinal tract and to remodel bone. PTH is involved in the differentiation and activation of osteoclasts to resorb bone. This is mediated indirectly by signals from the osteoblast (Chambers *et al.*, 1985). Similar effects are seen with 1,25 dihydroxy vitamin D_3, which can also inhibit T cell proliferation and production of IL-2.

8.7.2 Inflammatory cytokines

The most significant conceptual advance in bone pathology since the early 1980s was the realisation that many cytokines could act as autocrine and paracrine regulators of patho-physiological bone resorption. A major problem facing bone biologists today is the sheer numbers of cytokines and their complex mechanisms and interactions. This is a situation that can easily be described as chaotic in

Table 8.1 *The pathological and physiological regulators of bone resorption*

		Stimulators of bone resorption	Osteoclast differentiation/formation
Hormones			
Parathyroid hormone (PTH)		+	+
1,25-Dihydroxy vitamin D$_3$ (1,25 Vit D)		+	+
Glucocorticoids		+/−	+/−
Calcitonin (CT)		−	−
Cytokines			
Interleukins	IL-1	+	+
	IL-2	+/−	+/−
	IL-3	?	+
	IL-4	−	−
	IL-6	+/−	+
	IL-8	−	−
	IL-10	−	−
	IL-11	+	+
	IL-13	−	?
Tumour necrosis factor (TNFα)		+	+
Colony-stimulating factors	GM-CSF	+	+
	M-CSF	?	+
	LIF	+/−	+
	SCF	−	+
Interferon gamma (IFN-γ)		−	−
Growth factors			
Insulin like growth factors	IGF-I	+/−	+
	IGF-II	+/−	+
Transforming growth factor β (TGFβ)		+/−	+/−
Fibroblast growth factors	Acidic FGF	+	+
	Basic FGF	+	+
Platelet-derived growth factors	PDGF-AA	+	+
	PDGF-AB	+	+
	PDGF-BB	+	+
Epidermal growth factor (EGF)		+	+
Bone morphogenic proteins (BMPs 1–8)		+/−	+/−
Others			
Oestrogen		−	−
Heparin		+	?
Thyroid hormones		+	+
Bradykinin		+	+
Thrombin		+	?
Vitamin A		+	+
Prostaglandin E$_2$		+	+
Reactive O$_2$ and N$_2$ species			
Nitric oxide	˙NO	+/−	?
Superoxide	O$_2$˙$^-$	+/−	?
Hydrogen peroxide	H$_2$O$_2$	+	?
Peroxynitrite	ONOO$^-$	?	?

+, positive effects of bone resorption, differentiation and activation; −, negative effects; +/−, factors can stimulate or inhibit the bone resorptive process; ?, effects have yet to be elucidated.

pathological situations where cytokine responses are non-linear and interacting. This premise of non-linearity and interactive response drives the mathematics of chaos.

The initial discovery that the proinflammatory cytokines IL-1 and TNF could stimulate bone resorption led to several other cytokines being implicated in bone resorption (Bertolini *et al.*, 1986). Since the bone microenvironment contains cells that can produce many of these cytokines, it is possible that the action of one cytokine may be influenced by another. This appears to be the case for IL-6, which dramatically enhances bone resorption stimulated by IL-1 and TNF but does not stimulate bone resorption mediated by PTH and 1,25-dihydroxy vitamin D_3. Subsequent inhibition of IL-6 generation prevents IL-1 or TNF from inducing resorption of bone (Mundy, 1991). These data show the complex interactions that are occurring in the bone-resorbing environment between these cytokines. Currently, several cytokines and colony-stimulating factors have been implicated in the differentiation and development of osteoclasts and osteoblasts. This includes $TNF\alpha$, the interleukins IL-1, IL-3, IL-6 and IL-11, GM-CSF and M-CSF. The proinflammatory cytokines $TNF\alpha$ and $IL-1\beta$ mediate their osteoclastogenic actions via other factors derived from stromal/osteoblastic cells. Inhibitors of bone resorption appear to be IL-4, IL-8 and IFN-γ; the last is a multifunctional cytokine that can inhibit the proliferation and differentiation of osteoclast progenitors.

It is well documented that the cytokines $IL-1\beta$, $TNF\alpha$, IL-6 and M-CSF are elevated in the rheumatoid joint, whereas levels of IFN-γ and IL-2 have been found to be low. This unusual pattern of cytokine response may be linked to the hypoxic nature of the mobile inflamed joint. The extracellular matrix of bone is a rich source of growth factors, including $TGF\beta$, the FGFs, IGFs, PDGFs and BMPs, which are all implicated in the stimulation of new bone formation via the osteoblastic lineage. $TGF\beta$, a growth regulatory factor that is synthesized by many tissues including bone, inhibits osteoclast formation and differentiation. Since $TGF\beta$ is within the extracellular matrix, it may be an important factor in inhibiting osteoclastic activity and promoting bone formation. The problem in inflammatory arthritis is that increased levels of cytokines may outweigh the levels of growth factors released from the bone matrix, propagating the imbalance between resorption and formation.

8.7.3 Reactive oxygen–nitrogen species

The identity of local mediators produced by the osteoblast to activate the osteoclast has been the subject of much debate. Prostaglandins were thought to be this molecule because cytokines were able to induce prostaglandin synthesis by osteoblasts and prostaglandins were able to stimulate formation and activation of osteoclasts. However, there have been a variety of studies demonstrating that COX inhibitors, though able to block PGE_2 biosynthesis by $TNF\alpha$, are incapable or only partially able to inhibit bone resorption (Lerner and Ohlin, 1993). This indicates that there must be a prostaglandin-independent mechanism involved in cytokine-induced bone resorption. Cytokines have been shown to stimulate cells from the synovium and cartilage to produce both reactive oxygen and reactive nitrogen species (Ralston *et al.*, 1995). These metabolites also appear to be involved in the coupling of osteoblast/osteoclast bone resorption in a similar way to the coupling of endothelial and smooth muscle cells in relation to blood flow homeostasis.

8.8 What is unique about the environment within the inflamed joint?

A variety of studies of the metabolic characteristics of inflamed rheumatoid joints reveal that it is a chronically hypoxic environment. Synovial tissue analysed by nuclear magnetic resonance spectroscopy displays a profile of low-molecular-weight metabolites consistent with hypoxic metabolism (Naughton *et al.*, 1993). The main characteristics are a lowered glucose content and increased lactate. More recent studies utilizing a polarographic needle electrode have measured oxygen levels in synovium directly and have shown generally lower levels in rheumatoid knees, with pockets of tissue that are profoundly hypoxic. This is supported by the morphometric analysis of the inflamed synovial tissue, indicating inadequate perfusion owing to failure of angiogenesis to vascularize the innermost layer of synovium (Stevens *et al.*, 1991). In addition to this, movement of the inflamed joint results in pressure changes that lead to repeated cycles of ischaemia/reperfusion. The inflamed joint tissue is, therefore, exposed to the influences of hypoxia-induced events that can be modulated by the intermittent reperfusion, particularly in the subsynovium where the vasculature is more adequately developed. These characteristics create a unique redox-controlled environment within the inflamed synovium where both reducing (owing to chronic hypoxia) and oxidizing (owing to intermittent reperfusion) events prevail. Evidence for the existence of such an environment with differentially oxidizing and reducing components comes from the observations of high intracellular but low extracellular sulphydryl levels in the inflamed synovium. The presence of oxidatively modified extracellular biomolecules in synovitis also supports this observation.

8.9 How might hypoxia affect bone resorption?

During hypoxia, a complex series of events contribute to the creation of an environment where a functional compartmentalization of the subsynovium and the 'invasive' surface lining, or pannus, occurs. Because of the differential vascular distribution of these two compartments, it seems likely that the subsynovium is more prone to oxidative influences during reperfusion of the joint, leading to the persistence of the inflammatory reaction. In contrast, hypoxia-driven events play a greater role in the development of the pathology involving the pannus tissue, which abuts bare bone. Within the chronically hypoxic surface layer and within erosive sites, fibroblastic lining cells have a transformed morphology and respond by increased secretion of $\alpha(1)$ procollagen, procathepsin D and endonuclease. These changes particularly reflect dissolution of the basement membrane and migration and proliferation of fibroblasts into the underlying bone tissue, creating erosive damage. The expression of the SVL30 retroelement may be an indication of the reported adaptation of a transformed phenotype by fibroblasts, which would further contribute to this non-metastatic, hypoxia-driven invasion of the bone tissue. Induction of PDGF secretion and the anchorage-independent growth characteristics of these cells also support their unscheduled proliferative state. Moreover, transcriptional up-regulation of vascular endothelial growth factor (VEGF) expression in these cells in response to hypoxia also reflects an attempt to establish the much required perfusion by inducing angiogenesis. Many of these events are modulated by transcriptional induction of related genes as a consequence of activation and binding of a range of transcription factors (particularly hypoxia-inducible factor, HIF) to hypoxia-response elements (HRE) in their promoters. Perhaps, induction of the COX enzymes (particularly COX-2) during hypoxia (Schmedtje *et al.*, 1997) is one of the most important events that could provide an explanation for the ineffectiveness of NSAIDs on bone erosions in RA, where a significant benefit of NSAID treatment is seen on the synovitis. Within the subsynovium, hypoxically induced COX enzymes will function adequately on reperfusion, since oxygen is a required substrate and will contribute to the inflammatory reaction. Inhibition of these enzymes with NSAIDs will, thus, effectively limit the inflammatory component of the pathology. In contrast, although these enzymes will also be induced within the hypoxic pannus tissue, lack of adequate perfusion and associated lack of the substrate will limit their function. This, clearly limits the contribution of COX enzymes to the pannus-controlled bone resorption, where NSAIDs that inhibit COX-1 and COX-2 are ineffective. It also follows that delivery of drugs with high partition coefficients to poorly vascularized hypoxic tissues, such as synovial pannus, will not be effective in stopping bone damage.

Within the synovial tissue, cells of the macrophage/monocyte lineage respond to hypoxia by releasing an extensive catalogue of cytokines, including TNFα, IL-1 to IL-10 and TGFβ, which not only drive inflammation (Badolato and Oppenheim 1996) but also, as shown, mediate pathological bone resorption (Mundy, 1993). Endothelial cells respond by transcriptional induction or enhanced surface expression of a series of integrin molecules (endothelial leukocyte adhesion molecule 1/intercellular adhesion molecule 1 (ELAM-1/ICAM-1)), which mediate extravascular trafficking of lymphocytes and neutrophils and maintain the inflammatory reaction. Lymphocytes and neutrophils also show enhanced expression of the associated integrins (lymphocyte function associated antigen 1 (LFA-1), vascular cell adhesion molecule 1 (VCAM-1), very late antigen 4 (VLA-4) and CD11a/CD18) in response to hypoxia. The expression of these integrin molecules may induce the recruitment of inflammatory cells with a repertoire of proresorptive cytokines under hypoxia. In inflamed synovial tissues, T lymphocytes show a predominant T$_H$1 cytokine pattern under conditions of hypoxia, but IL-2 levels are low (Zuckerberg, Goldberg and Lederman, 1994).

Hypoxia and hypoxia-induced cytokines such as TNFα and IL-1 transcriptionally induce the expression of two enzymes we believe to be instrumental in the osteoblast–osteoclast uncoupling that leads to bone resorption. These are iNOS and xanthine oxidoreductase (XOR). The role of these two enzymes in the bone resorption associated with rheumatoid disease is discussed below.

8.10 How oxidants affect biological systems

Cellular responses to oxidants are diverse. The nature of these responses is not only dependent on the extent of oxidative stress but also on the intrinsic anti-oxidant status of different cell types. Therefore, differential 'oxidant sensitivity' is observed within different cell populations. The involvement of oxidants such as hydrogen peroxide and NO in processes as diverse as apoptosis, stress protein response and proliferation, for example, clearly reflects the complexity of their interactions. Although complex, and with largely unknown mechanisms of action, these oxidants are known to act as signalling molecules. Oxidant-mediated induction of the growth competence genes c-*myc*, c-*fos*, and c-*jun* is well documented. The significant role of the c-*fos* oncogene in the regulation of bone remodelling infers potential modulation of related processes by oxidants. Furthermore, the c-*src* proto-onco-gene, known to play a critical role in the development of ruffled border in osteoclasts for resorptive activity, is also activated by oxidant-mediated phosphor-ylation of its associated protein product pp60^{src}. Two transcription factors, AP-1 and NF-κB, are also oxidant sensitive. Collagenase and stromelysin genes both have AP-1-binding elements in their promoter regions, which thus confers oxidant sensitivity to these genes integral to the bone matrix dissolution process. Oxidant-sensitive AP-1 also mediates the transcriptional activation of resorption-modulating cytokine genes such as those for TGFβ and IL-2.

Oxidant-mediated modulation of the gene for osteopontin, which is integral in several processes involving bone remodelling (mineralization, cell attachment and migration), and the hypoxia-response element on iNOS gene (iNOS-HRE) have also been reported. Oxidants also mediate the activation of the transcription factor NF-κB. NF-κB regulates the transcription of a multitude of proresorptive cytokine genes, including TNFα, IL-1, IL-6, IL-8 and GM-CSF. In addition, the adhesion molecules E-selectin and VCAM-1, the acute-phase proteins angiotensinogen and serum amyloid A precursor as well as the poliferation-linked proto-oncogene c-*myc* are target genes for NF-κB, reflecting its role in the maintenance of the inflamma-tory reaction as well as in bone resorptive processes.

In summary, hypoxia- and hypoxia/reperfusion-mediated disruption of cellular interactions, either at the level of the intrinsic anti-oxidants or at the level of the anti-oxidant/oxidant-responsive transcription factors, may lead to the dysregulation of physiologically coordinated processes such as bone remodelling (Figure 8.2). Such disturbances in this finely tuned phenomenon of oxidant/anti-oxidant balance may be the underlying reason for both chronic inflammation and uncontrolled bone resorption in RA. We hypothesize that the enzyme systems xanthine oxidoreductase and iNOS play a key role in these processes.

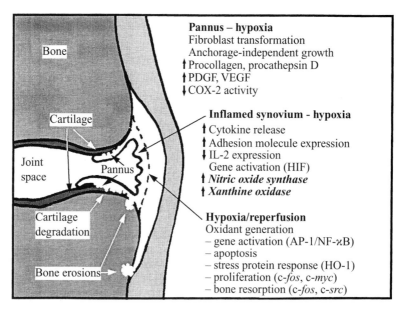

Figure 8.2 Summary of hypoxia- and hypoxia/reperfusion-induced events in inflamed synovium, which, we propose, modulate bone resorption.

8.11 The environment of resorbing bone

The production of superoxide or other reactive oxygen species by activated osteoclasts is implicated in the complex process of bone resorption. The mineral and organic phases of bone are degraded in Howship's lacunae. These are sealed compartments formed by the integrin-mediated adhesion of osteoclast basal membrane to the mineralized bone surface. The lacunae are highly acidic, an environment conducive to the degradation of the mineral phase of the bone, predominantly crystalline hydroxyapatite. The organic phase is degraded by a battery of osteoclast-derived proteolytic enzymes, including cathepsins, cysteine proteinases and matrix metalloproteinases. It is interesting to note that all of the above factors (integrin up-regulation, acidosis and proteolytic enzyme activation) are initiated or enhanced by a hypoxic environment.

8.12 Radicals, hypoxia and bone resorption

How do reactive oxygen species influence these processes? The answer is predictably complex but we can begin to unravel the problem based on recently published work. There are several levels at which reactive oxygen species may be involved. Superoxide is known to be generated via NADPH oxidase in the ruffled border (osteoclastic margin of the resorption lacuna) and released into the site of resorption. Superoxide dismutase can inhibit resorption at this level, implying that the degradation of the matrix itself may be enhanced by oxidative damage caused by superoxide or oxidizing derivatives thereof.

There are several steps in the process leading up to the initiation of resorption activity by the osteoclast. These also appear to be somewhat under the control of reactive oxygen species. Osteoclasts, which are blood-borne multinucleated giant cells from the same haematopoietic mononuclear stem cell lineage as macrophages, have to be recruited and differentiated in the process of osteoclastogenesis. It has been shown that hydrogen peroxide, a product of superoxide dismutation but also generated directly by many cell types, can induce osteoclastogenesis and osteoclast motility *in vitro*. Fully differentiated osteoclasts have the potential to resorb bone, but only after appropriate stimulation. We have reviewed above the factors that are known to induce bone resorption, and it is clear that this is a diverse group. However, they have in common the requirement for their effect to be mediated via the osteoblast. It is widely held that in response to stimulation, osteoblasts induce osteoclastic bone resorption by secreting into the medium a small, soluble, labile factor (McSheehy and Chambers, 1987). These are the characteristics of reactive oxygen species and other free radicals such as NO, also implicated in bone resorptive processes (Chapters 10–12 and 16). Hydrogen peroxide, in fact, as well as increasing osteoclast number may be unique in its ability to activate osteoclasitc bone resorption directly in the absence of osteoblasts or other proresorptive stimuli (Bax *et al.*, 1992). Osteoblasts generate hydrogen peroxide directly in response to cytokines but it is also formed by the action of superoxide dismutase on superoxide, which is also generated in the resorption environment. Interestingly, a novel, developmentally regulated 150 kDa plasma membrane glycoprotein related to cytosolic Mn^{2+} superoxide dismutase has been reported on osteoclasts and identified as the ligand for the osteoclast-specific monoclonal antibody (MAb) 121F. This superoxide dismutase-related membrane component may serve as a signal-transducing molecule at the osteoclast surface, converting osteoblast- or osteoclast-derived superoxide to hydrogen peroxide, since its functional blockade using Fab fragments of MAb 121F inhibit in a dose-dependent manner osteoclastic bone particle and pit resorption activity (Oursler, Li and Osdoby, 1991).

8.13 Bone-derived reactive oxygen species

What is the source of these reactive oxygen species in bone? There may be more than one answer, but the ideal candidate should be controllable and sensitive to those stimuli which have been identified as proresorptive. We have considered the strongest candidate to be the enzyme xanthine oxidoreductase. This is a cytosolic and membrane-bound complex molybdoflavoprotein with two Fe–S clusters; it is a constitutive enzyme involved in the purine metabolism of most cells. During the catalysis of xanthine to uric acid, xanthine oxidoreductase can use NAD^+ (dehydrogenase form) or molecular oxygen (oxidase form) as an electron acceptor. The oxidase form, therefore, generates the superoxide anion radical and hydrogen peroxide and is a candidate for the source of these communication signals. The gene for human xanthine oxidoreductase has been cloned and investigated (Xu, Huecksteadt and Hoidal, 1996). It is located on chromosome 2 at band p22 and contains two transcriptional initiation sites consisting of sequences coding for a number of promoter elements associated with the acute-phase response genes. These included four CAAT/enhancer binding protein sites, three IL-6 regulatory elements, an NF-κB site and five IFN-γ responsive elements. Other than these inflammation-related promoters, the gene also contains an AP-1 motif, three potential AP-2 sites, a potential responsive element for glucocorticoid hormone regulation and a putative HIF-1-binding site. The last factor may explain the observed up-regulation of xanthine oxidoreductase by hypoxia in a variety of cell types. It can also be seen that the control of the xanthine oxidoreductase gene itself may be influenced by the oxidants generated by the enzyme, in the ways described above. The analysis of the gene also identifies potential mechanisms for its up-regulation by the inflammatory cytokines TNFα and IL-1β in various cells. These cytokines are established inducers of bone resorption both *in vitro* and *in vivo* and it can be construed that their abundance in rheumatoid joints may facilitate the destruction of joints by bone erosion. TNFα up-regulates the mRNA, protein levels and activity of xanthine oxidoreductase in rat osteoblasts. Our recent work has established a possible mechanism of cytokine-induced *in vitro* bone resorption involving the stimulatory influence of hydrogen peroxide generated by xanthine oxidoreductase. The capacity for hydrogen peroxide generation by xanthine oxido-reductase is increased by TNFα in osteoblasts; the proresorptive effect of TNFα and IL-1β can be blocked either by scavenging hydrogen peroxide with catalase or by blocking its generation using competitive and non-competitive xanthine oxidor-eductase inhibitors. This mechanism certainly applies *in vitro* and may well constitute a major part of *in vivo* pathological bone resorption.

8.14 NO

The *in vivo* situation is of course much more complex and is influenced by many and variable factors reacting and interacting in the bone environment. One major influence that may bear relevance to our hypothesis is the role of NO in bone resorption. Proresorptive cytokines also up-regulate iNOS in osteoblasts and hence increase NO generation by these cells. In fact, the iNOS gene shares many of the promoter characteristics of the xanthine oxidoreductase gene. Small, induced concentrations of NO appear to be necessary for bone resorption, whereas high levels resulting from superinduction of iNOS have an inhibitory effect.

8.15 The peroxynitrite factor

The interaction of NO and superoxide is important in controlling the individual effects of either in biological systems. It seems reasonable to suggest that osteoblastic control of bone resorption is dependent upon a balance of these two radical species. Superoxide reacts extremely rapidly with NO to form another powerful oxidant, the peroxynitrite anion ($ONOO^-$). Peroxynitrite is cytotoxic and its biological actions are deleterious and exacerbated during disease and inflammation. Although peroxynitrite can oxidize many biomolecules, in biological systems it reacts mostly with carbon dioxide to form one or more intermediates that are oxidants and nitrating agents. The hydroxyl radical was once thought to be an end point in the degradation of peroxynitrite, but it has now been shown to form a metastable intermediate that is more selective than the hydroxyl radical and, therefore, can reach more distant sites. It is not known what the effect of peroxynitrite is on bone resorption or whether the observed, supposed effects of O_2^- and NO are in fact caused by peroxynitrite, since inhibiting either of these species will also reduce peroxynitrite concentration.

8.16 Coupling/uncoupling

Considering that the osteoblast contains both iNOS and xanthine oxidoreductase and that these enzymes may be differentially controlled or expressed by a complex assortment of 'bone resorptive' factors, there is a high likelihood that peroxynitrite will be present in the resorbing environment. As alluded to above, these considerations allow the possibility that the physiological coupling of osteoblasts and osteoclasts by reactive oxygen and nitrogen species in bone remodelling could, under altered environmental conditions such as exist under hypoxic invading pannus, result in the uncoupling of the system in pathological, erosive situations such as RA. The implications of this will be a subject for further concerted investigation. The roles we propose for reactive oxygen and nitrogen species on bone resorption are schematically represented in Figure 8.3.

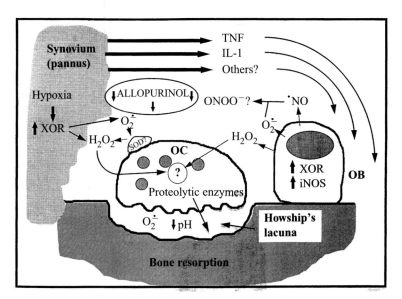

Figure 8.3 Oxidative influences on rheumatoid bone erosions. Xanthine oxidoreductase (XOR) is a source of oxidants from the cells in the synovium and from osteoblasts (OB). We propose, based on our *in vitro* studies, that the influence of these oxidants on the osteoclast (OC) can be inhibited by allopurinol.

References

Badolato, R. and Oppenheim J. J. (1996) Role of cytokines acute-phase proteins, and chemokines in the progression of rhuematoid arthritis. *Sem. Arthritis Rheum.* **26**, 526–538.

Bax, B. E., Alam, A. S., Banerji, B. *et al.* (1992) Stimulation of osteoclastic bone resorption by hydrogen peroxide. *Biochem. Biophys. Res. Commun.* **183**, 1153–1158.

Bertolini, D. R., Nedwin, G. E., Bringman, T. S., Smith, D. and Mundy, G. R. (1986) Stimulation of bone resorption and inhibition of bone formation *in vitro* by human tumour necrosis factors. *Nature* **319**, 516–518.

Bilezikian, J. P., Raisz, L. G. and Rodan G. A. (eds) (1996) *Principles of Bone Biology.* Academic Press, San Diego, USA.

Chambers, T. J., McSheehy, P. M. J., Thomson, B. M.and Fuller, K. (1985) The effect of calcium-regulating hormones, prostaglandins, on bone resorption by osteoclasts disaggregated from neonatal rabbit bones. *Endocrinology* **116**, 234–239.

Kidd, B. L., Cruwys, S. and Polak, J. M. (1990) Neurogenic mechanism for symmetrical arthritis [letter]. *Lancet* **335**, 795.

Kirwan, J. R. (1995) The effect of glucocorticoids on joint destruction in rheumatoid arthritis. The Arthritis and Rheumatism Council Low-Dose Glucocorticoid Study Group. *N. Engl. J. Med.* **333**, 142–146.

Lerner, U. H. and Ohlin, A. (1993) Tumour necrosis factors a and b can stimulate bone resorption in cultured mouse calvariae by a prostaglandin-independent mechanism. *J. Bone Min. Res.* **8**, 147–155.

McSheehy, P. M. and Chambers, T. J. (1987) 1,25-Dihydroxyvitamin D_3 stimulates rat osteoblastic cells to release a soluble factor that increases osteoclastic bone resorption. *J. Clin. Invest.* **80**, 425–429.

Mundy, G. R. (1991) Inflammatory mediators and the destruction of bone. *J. Periodontol. Res.* **26**, 213–217.

Mundy, G. R. (1993) Cytokines and growth factors in the regulation of bone remodelling. *J. Bone Min. Res.* **8**, (Suppl. 2), S505–S510.

Naughton, D. P., Haywood, R., Blake, D. R., Edmonds, S., Hawkes, G. E. and Grootveld, M. (1993) A comparative evaluation of the metabolic profiles of normal and inflammatory knee-joint synovial fluids by high resolution proton NMR spectroscopy. *FEBS Lett.* **332**, 221–225.

Oursler, M. J., Li, L. and Osdoby, P. (1991) Purification and characterisation of an osteoclast membrane glycoprotein with homology to manganese superoxide dismutase. *J. Cell Biochem.* **46**, 219–233.

Ralston, S. H., Ho, L. P., Helfrich, M. H., Grabowski, P. S., Johnston, P. W. and Benjamin, N. (1995) Nitric oxide: a cytokine-induced regulator of bone resorption. *J. Bone Min. Res.* **10**, 1040–1049.

Resnick, D., Bernthiaume, M.-S. and Sartoris, D. (1993) Imaging. In *Textbook of Rheumatology,* 4th edn. (ed. W. Kelley, E. Harris, S. Ruddy and B. Sledge), pp. 579–629. W. B. Saunders, Philadelphia, PA.

Schmedtje, J. F. Jr, Ji, Y. S., Liu, W. L., DuBois, R. N. and Runge, M. S. (1997) Hypoxia induces cyclo-oxygenase-2 via the NF-kappaB p65 transcription factor in human vascular endothelial cells. *J. Biol. Chem.* **272**, 601–608.

Stevens, C. R., Blake, D. R., Merry, P., Revell, P. A. and Levick, J. R. (1991) A comparative study by morphometry of the microvasculature in normal and rheumatoid synovium. *Arthritis Rheum.* **34**, 1508–1513.

Xu, P., Huecksteadt, T. P. and Hoidal, J. R. (1996) Molecular cloning and characterisation of the human xanthine dehydrogenase gene (XDH). *Genomics* **34**, 173–180.

Zuckerberg, A. L., Goldberg, L. I. and Lederman, H. M. (1994) Effects of hypoxia on interleukin-2 mRNA expression by T lymphocytes. *Crit. Care Med.* **22**, 197–203.

9

Nitric oxide and cartilage matrix turnover

MIN CAO, HANS-JORG HÄUSELMANN, MAJA
STEFANOVIC-RACIC and CHRISTOPHER H. EVANS

9.1 Introduction

Following activation by the appropriate cytokines, chondrocytes make as much, if not more, NO than any other cell in the body. This fact alone suggests than NO is very important in the metabolism of activated chondrocytes. Data in support of this conclusion are beginning to accumulate, although, as is typical for studies of NO, the story is not a straightforward one and contradictions exist within the literature. The key question of whether pharmacological manipulation of NO activity will prove useful in diseases affecting cartilage remains unanswered. In this chapter, we review what is presently known about these matters (see Evans, Watkins and Stafanovic-Racic (1996) for recent review).

9.2 NO production by cartilage

All cartilage tissues yet examined, including articular cartilage (Stadler *et al.*, 1991), costal cartilage (Kondo *et al.*, 1993) and intervertebral disc (Kang *et al.*, 1995), produce large amounts of NO following treatment with the appropriate inducing factors. Unlike certain other cell types, high levels of NO are generated by human (Palmer *et al.*, 1993), as well as rodent chondrocytes. Murrell *et al.* (1996a) have reported that meniscal cartilage lacks this ability, but we have been able to induce the synthesis of copious amounts of NO by cultures of lapine (Cao *et al.*, 1998) and human (M. Cao *et al.*, unpublished data) meniscus.

In general, NO production by normal, unactivated tissue remains below the limit of detection. For high levels of NO production, it is necessary to retrieve the tissue from sites of disease, or to culture the tissue in the presence of cytokines; a recent report indicates that chondrocytes also increase their production of NO in response to shear (Das, Schurman and Lane Smith, 1997). Chondrocytes are unusual in their ability to synthesize large quantities of NO in response to a single cytokine. IL-1 is often used for this purpose, but chondrocytes also respond to TNFα, leukaemia inhibitory factor (LIF) and IL-17 (Rediske *et al.*, 1994; Lotz *et al.*, 1996). Chondrocytes are also unusual in that NO production is not inhibited by

TGFβ, which for most other types of cell is a very potent down-regulator of NO synthesis.

The foregoing discussion suggests that chondrocytes do not possess either of the constitutive forms of NOS but they do express an inducible NOS. Molecular analysis bears this out (Charles *et al.*, 1993). It has not been possible to detect mRNAs encoding eNOS or nNOS in either resting or activated chondrocytes isolated from normal human joints (Maier *et al.*, 1994). The latter, however, express mRNA encoding iNOS (Charles *et al.*, 1993; Maier *et al.*, 1994). Amin *et al.* (1995) have presented evidence that the NOS present in human articular chondrocytes recovered from osteoarthritic joints is aberrant. They suggest that these cells express high levels of a dysregulated nNOS, although the possibility that this is a novel isoform of NOS (OA-NOS) has been actively discussed. When Grabowski and co-workers (Grabowski, MacPherson and Ralston, 1996) placed human articular chondrocytes into cell culture and stimulated them with cytokines, only transcripts encoding iNOS were identified. The issue of OA-NOS awaits clarification. The induction of NOS in chondrocytes is also atypical in its resistance to steroids (Palmer *et al.*, 1992). Another puzzling observation is that NO production by chondrocytes peaks 1–2 days after incubation and then rapidly falls to a much lower level (Stefanovic-Racic *et al.*, 1996a, 1997).

Recent studies on bovine (Fukuda *et al.*, 1995; Hayashi *et al.*, 1997) and human (Häuselmann *et al.*, 1998) articular cartilage have demonstrated that the superficial cells produce much more NO per cell in response to IL-1 than the deep cells. This is consistent with the observation that superficial cells are much more responsive to IL-1, possibly because they contain more type 1 IL-1 receptors.

9.3 Effects of NO on cartilage matrix turnover

In general physiological terms, the two most important functions of chondrocytes are to synthesize and to degrade the extracellular matrix. When these two activities are discordant, there are pathological consequences. Initial studies to identify a role for endogenously produced NO in cartilage metabolism, therefore, focused on matrix turnover.

There is almost unanimous agreement that endogenously produced NO inhibits the synthesis of proteoglycans by articular chondrocytes. The only exception is bovine articular cartilage, which, for some reason, lacks this response (Stefanovic-Racic *et al.*, 1996b). Nevertheless, in all other species that have yet been tested, including rabbits (Taskiran *et al.*, 1994), rats (Jarvinen *et al.*, 1995), mice (J. S. Mudgett, personal communication) and humans (Häuselmann *et al.*, 1994), NO strongly supresses the incorporation of $^{35}SO_4^{2-}$ into cartilage proteoglycans. The unresponsiveness of bovine tissue is not because bovine articular chondrocytes fail to produce NO; like the chondrocytes of other species, they are capable of synthesizing very large amounts of this radical (Stefanovic-Racic *et al.*, 1996a). The mechanism through which NO inhibits proteoglycan synthesis is not known, but our preliminary data suggest an effect on the synthesis of the core protein rather than on the synthesis of glycosaminoglycans (Stefanovic-Racic *et al.*, 1998).

Endogenously produced NO also inhibits the synthesis of collagen by articular (Cao *et al.*, 1997) and meniscal (Cao *et al.*, 1998) cartilage without greatly altering the synthesis of non-collagenous proteins. In neither tissue is there a major effect on the abundance of the mRNAs encoding the α chains of the various collagens. This suggests that NO inhibits collagen synthesis at a translational or a post-translational level. There is preliminary evidence that NO inhibits prolyl hydro-xylase, an important enzyme in the post-translational processing of collagen (Cao *et al.*, 1997). The mechanism of this inhibition is under investigation.

It has been widely assumed that NO would be a mediator of matrix catabolism. However, detailed *in vitro* studies using slices of bovine (Stefanovic-Racic *et al.*, 1996a) and lapine (Stefanovic-Racic *et al.*, 1997) articular cartilage, as well as alginate cultures of human articular chondrocytes (Häuselmann *et al.*, 1998), have not borne this out. Instead, the data suggest that, if anything, NO is protective. Analysis of the conditioned media recovered during the study of bovine and lapine tissue revealed higher levels of matrix metalloproteinases (MMPs) when NO synthesis was blocked. This suggests that NO suppresses MMP production and provides a mechanism for its apparent chondroprotective effect. However, other studies suggest that NO enhances MMP production (Murrell, Jang and Williams, 1996b). The reason for this discrepancy is unknown, but it is worth noting that inhibition of MMP production was found using slices of otherwise intact cartilage, whereas stimulation of MMP production was found in monolayer culture. Chondrocytes are notorious for the ease with which they dedifferentiate under the latter culture conditions.

9.4 Effects of NO on chondrocyte metabolism

There is increasing appreciation of the importance of autocrine agents, such as NO, in the regulation of chondrocyte metabolism. Many of these autocrine agents regulate each other's activities in a complex, interwoven fashion. NO appears to be no exception. As shown in Table 9.1, NO inhibits the production of a variety of cytokines, particularly IL-6, by chondrocytes (Evans *et al.*, 1994). The significance of IL-6 inhibition, which has also been shown for human invertebral disc (Kang *et al.*, 1995), is difficult to assess because the role of IL-6 in cartilage metabolism is unknown.

The literature contains contradictory reports on the effect of NO on PGE$_2$ production (Table 9.1). We have shown that NO strongly suppresses PGE$_2$ produc-tion by lapine (Stadler *et al.*, 1991) and human (Evans *et al.*, 1994) chondrocytes. Amin and co-workers (1997) recently confirmed this and suggested a mechanism whereby NO inhibits the induction of COX-2 by preventing the activation of the transcription factor NF-κB. Two other reports, however, suggest that NO increases PGE$_2$ production by increasing the activity of COX (Blanco and Lotz, 1995; Marfield, Jang and Murrell, 1996). Such a response would be consistent with the

Table 9.1. *Effect of NO on production of cytokines and PGE$_2$ by articular chondrocytes*

Mediator	Effect of NO[a]	Reference
IL-6	−	Evans *et al.*, 1994
IL-8	−	Our unpublished data
IL-1 ra	−	Evans *et al.*, 1994; Pelletier *et al.*, 1996
PGE$_2$	−	Stadler *et al.*, 1991; Evans *et al.*, 1994; Amin *et al.*, 1997
	+	Blanco *et al.*, 1995; Marfield *et al.*, 1996

[a] NO inhibits, −; stimulates, +.

literature on other types of cell, where a stimulatory effect has been widely reported. The disagreement in the literature concerning chondrocytes may again come down to culture conditions, as the two reports indicating a stimulatory effect of NO upon PGE$_2$ production utilized monolayer cultures. This matter is not merely academic, as PGE$_2$ influences matrix metabolism in important ways and has been held responsible for the inhibition of chondrocyte cell division by NO (Blanco and Lotz, 1995).

NO also inhibits chondrocyte migration and adhesion to fibronectin, possibly by interfering with the assembly of the cytoskeleton (Frenkel *et al.*, 1996). This, and its ability to inhibit matrix production, suggest that NO reduces the ability of chondrocytes to repair cartilaginous lesions.

Another factor could be cell death. Blanco and co-workers suggest that NO causes apoptosis in articular chondrocytes (Blanco *et al.*, 1995). According to these authors, whether or not cells die depends upon the production of other reactive oxygen species by the cells. The latter, such as superoxide and hydrogen peroxide, provoke cell death by necrosis. If NO and the reactive oxygen species are produced together, they neutralize each other and the cells survive. This is clearly an important concept and raises the issue of the degree to which chondrocytes produce other radical species, such as superoxide. It is well known that NO and superoxide combine rapidly to generate peroxynitrite (ONOO$^-$), a molecule that nitrosylates aromatic amino acids such as tyrosine and which is held responsible for a number of biological effects that were previously ascribed to NO.

NO also influences the energy metabolism of chondrocytes. It promotes the production of large amounts of lactic acid and may compromise the production of ATP (Stefanovic-Racic *et al.*, 1994). This could be the relevance to the suppression of matrix synthesis, which is known to be sensitive to the cell's energy charge (Baker, Feigan and Lauther, 1989).

9.5 Production of NO in arthritis

Ex vivo examination of articular cartilage recovered from the joints of patients with osteoarthritis and RA has confirmed the expression of NOS in these diseases

(Sakurai *et al.*, 1995). Antibodies and antisense probes to iNOS protein and mRNA, respectively, were used in these analyses, suggesting that the isoform of NOS expressed in these tissues is indeed iNOS. However, until there is resolution of the matter of OA-NOS, discussed earlier in this chapter, final judgement should be withheld.

Normal articular cartilage did not contain message or protein for NOS, suggesting that this enzyme is induced during the disease process. The question is, at what stage? For practical reasons, the tissues examined in these studies were obtained at the time of total joint replacement, which means that the joints had end-stage disease. Because of this, there was ample opportunity for secondary changes. It will be important to know at what state NOS is induced during the onset and progression of the different forms of arthritis.

The presence of NOS within chondrocytes recovered from arthritic joints does not automatically mean that NO was being made. We have measured *ex vivo* NO production by human cartilage (Stefanovic-Racic *et al.*, 1996b). Although NO synthesis by osteoarthritic cartilage is elevated compared with normal, it is only about 25% of the levels produced by the same samples after treatment with IL-1. This is reminiscent of the levels produced by chondrocytes after chronic exposure to IL-1 *in vitro*. It supports the suggestion that NO production by chondrocytes in arthritis persists chronically at a slightly elevated level, with high levels of production occurring episodically in conjunction with flares or other such disturbances.

9.6 Conclusions

Underlying studies of the type described in this chapter is the idea that modulation of NO activity in cartilage will be beneficial in arthritis. Until the role of NO in cartilage metabolism is defined more precisely, however, this remains speculative.

Acknowledgement

The authors' work in this area has been supported by NIH grant number AR42025. Lou Duerring kindly typed the manuscript.

References

Amin, A. R., DiCesare, P. E., Vyas, P. *et al.* (1995) The expression and regulation of nitric oxide synthase in human osteoarthritis-affected chondrocytes: evidence for up-regulated neuronal nitric oxide synthase. *J. Exp. Med* **182**, 2097–2102.

Amin, A. R., Attur, M., Patel, R. N. *et al.* (1997) Superinduction of cyclooxygenase-2 activity in human osteoarthritis affected cartilage. Influence of nitric oxide. *J. Clin. Invest.* **99**, 1231–1237.

Baker, M. S., Feigan, J. and Lauther, D. A. (1989) The mechanism of chondrocyte hydrogen peroxide damage. Depletion of intracellular ATP due to suppression of glycolysis caused by oxidation of glyceraldehyde-3-phosphate dehydrogenase. *J. Rheumatol.* **16**, 7–14.

Blanco, F. J. and Lotz, M. (1995) IL-1-induced nitric oxide inhibits chondrocyte proliferation via PGE$_2$. *Exp. Cell Res.* **218**, 319–325.

Blanco, F. J., Ochs, R. L., Schwartz, H. and Lotz, M. (1995) Chondrocyte apoptosis induced by nitric oxide. *Am. J. Pathol.* **146**, 75–86.

Cao, M., Stefanovic-Racic, M., Georgescu, H. I., Miller, L. A. and Evans, C. H. (1998) Generation of nitric oxide by lapine meniscal cells and its effects on collagen biosynthesis: stimulation of collagen production by arganine. *J. Orthop. Res.* in press.

Cao, M., Westerhausen-Larson, A., Niyibizi, C. *et al.* (1997) Nitric oxide inhibits the synthesis of type II collagen without altering Col2A1 mRNA abundance; prolyl hydroxylase as a possible target. *Biochem. J.* **324**, 305–310.

Charles, I. G., Palmer, R. M. J., Hickery, M. S. *et al.* (!993) Cloning, characterization, and expression of a cDNA encoding an inducible nitric oxide synthase from the human chondrocyte. *Proc. Natl. Acad. Sci., USA* **90**, 11 419–11 423.

Das, P., Schurman, D. J. and Lane Smith, R. (1997) Nitric oxide and G proteins mediate the response of bovine articular chondrocytes to fluid-induced shear. *J. Orthop. Res.* **15**, 87–93.

Evans, C. H., Oppliger, L., Michel, B. A. *et al.* (1994) Effect of nitric oxide on cytokine and prostaglandin synthesis by human articular cartilage. *Osteoarthritis Cart.* **2**(suppl. 1), 51.

Evans, C. H., Watkins, S. C. and Stefanovic-Racic, M. (1996) Nitric oxide and cartilage metabolism. *Meth. Enzymol.* **269**, 75–88.

Frenkel, S. R., Clancy, R. M., Ricci, R. L., DiCesare, P. E., Rediske, J. J. and Abramson, S. B. (1996) Effects of nitric oxide on chondrocyte migration, adhesion and cytoskeletal assembly. *Arthritis Rheum.* **39**, 1905–1912.

Fukuda, K., Kumano, F., Takayama, M., Saito, M., Otani, K. and Tanaka, S. (1995) Zonal differences in nitric oxide synthesis by bovine chondrocytes exposed to interleukin-1. *Inflamm. Res.* **44**, 434–437.

Grabowski, P. S., Macpherson, H. and Ralston, S. H. (1996) Nitric oxide production in cells derived from the human joint. *Br. J. Rheumatol.* **35**, 207–212.

Häuselmann, H. J., Oppliger, L., Michel, B. A., Stefanovic-Racic, M. and Evans, C. H. (1994) Nitric oxide and proteoglycan biosynthesis by human articular chondrocytes in alginate culture. *FEBS Lett.* **352**, 361–364.

Häuselmann, H. J., Stefanovic-Racic, M., Michel, B. A. and Evans, C. H. (1998) Differences in nitric oxide production by superficial and deep human articular chondrocytes: implications for proteoglycan turnover in inflammatory joint diseases. *J. Immunol.* **160**, 1444–1448.

Hayashi, T., Abe, E., Yamata, T., Taguchi, Y. and Jasin, H. E. (1997) Nitric oxide production by superficial and deep articular chondrocytes. *Arthritis Rheum.* **40**, 251–269.

Jarvinen, T. A. H., Moilanen, T., Jarvinen, T. L. N. and Moilanen, E. (1995) Nitric oxide mediates interleukin-1 induced inhibition of glycosaminoglycan synthesis in rat articular cartilage. *Med. Inflamm.* **4**, 107–111.

Kang, J. D., Georgescu, H. I., McIntyre-Larkin, L., Stefanovic-Racic, M. and Evans, C. H. (1995) Herniated cervical intervertebral discs spontaneously produce matrix metalloproteinases, nitric oxide, interleukin-6, and prostaglandin E$_2$. *Spine* **20**, 2373–2378.

Kondo, S., Ishiguro, N., Iwata, H., Nakashima, I. and Isobe, K. I. (1993) The effects of nitric oxide on chondrocytes and lymphocytes. *Biochem. Biophys. Res. Commun.* **197**, 1431–1437.

Lotz, M., Bober, L., Narula, S. and Dudler, J. (1996) IL-17 promotes cartilage degradation (abstract). *Arthritis Rheum.* **39**(suppl), S120 (Abst. 559).

Maier, R., Bilbe, G., Rediske, J. and Lotz, M. (1994) Inducible nitric oxide synthase from human articular chondrocytes: cDNA cloning and analysis of mRNA expression. *Biochim. Biophys. Acta* **1208**, 145–150.

Marfield, L., Jang, D. and Murrell, G. A. C. (1996) Nitric oxide enhances cyclooxygenase activity in articular cartilage. *Inflamm. Res.* **45**, 254–258.

Murrell, G. A. C., Dolan, M. M., Jang, D., Szabo, C., Warren, R. F. and Hannafin, J. A.

(1996a) Nitric oxide: an important articular free radical. *J. Bone Joint Surg.* **78A**, 265–274.

Murrell, G. A. C., Jang, D. and Williams, R. J. (1996b) Nitric oxide activates metalloprotease enzymes in articular cartilage. *Biochem. Biophys. Res. Commun.* **206**, 15–21.

Palmer, R. M. J., Andrews, T., Foxwell, N. A. and Moncada, S. (1992) Glucocorticoids do not affect the induction of a novel calcium-dependent nitric oxide synthase in rabbit chondrocytes. *Biochem. Biophys. Res. Commun.* **188**, 209–215.

Palmer, R. M. J., Hickery, M. S., Charles, I. G., Moncada, S. and Bayliss, M. T. (1993) Induction of nitric oxide synthase in human chondrocytes. *Biochem. Biophys. Res. Commun.* **193**, 398–405.

Pelletier, J. P., Mineau, F., Ranger, P., Tardif, G., Martel-Pelletier, J. (1996) The increased synthesis of inducible nitric oxide inhibits IL-1ra synthesis by human articular chondrocytes: possible role in osteoarthritic cartilage degradation. *Osteoarthritis Cart.* **4**, 77–84.

Rediske, J., Koehne, C., Zhang, B. and Lotz, M. (1994) The inducible production of nitric oxide by articular cell types. *Osteoarthritis Cart.* **2**, 199–206.

Sakurai, H., Kohsaka, H., Liu, M. F. *et al.* (1995) Nitric oxide production and inducible nitric oxide synthase expression in inflammatory arthritides. *J. Clin. Invest.* **96**, 2357–2363.

Stadler, J., Stefanovic-Racic, M., Billiar, T. R. *et al.* (1991) Articular chondrocytes synthesize nitric oxide in response to cytokines and lipopolysaccharide. *J. Immunol.* **147**, 3915–3920.

Stefanovic-Racic, M., Stadler, J., Georgescu, H. I. and Evans, C. H. (1994) Nitric oxide and energy production in articular chondrocytes. *J. Cell. Physiol.* **159**, 274–280.

Stefanovic-Racic, M., Morales, T. I., Taskiran, D., McIntyre, L. A. and Evans, C. H. (1996a) The role of nitric oxide in proteoglycan turnover by bovine articular cartilage organ cultures. *J. Immunol.* **156**, 1213–1220.

Stefanovic-Racic, M., Watkins, S. C., Kang, R., Turner, D. and Evans, C. H. (1996b) Identification of inducible nitric oxide synthase in human osteoarthritic cartilage. *Trans. Orthop. Res. Soc.* **21**, 534.

Stefanovic-Racic, M., Möllers, M., Miller, L. A. and Evans, C. H. (1997) Nitric oxide and proteoglycan turnover in rabbit articular cartilage. *J. Orthop. Res.* **15**, 422–429.

Stefanovic-Racic, M., Taskiran, D., Hering, T. M., Georgescu, H. I. and Evans, C. H. (1998) Nitric oxide inhibits synthesis of aggrecan core protein without altering RNA abundance. *Trans. Orthop. Res. Soc.* **23**, 300.

Taskiran, D., Stefanovic-Racic, M., Georgescu, H. I. and Evans, C. H. (1994) Nitric oxide mediates suppression of cartilage proteoglycan synthesis by interleukin-1. *Biochem. Biophys. Res. Commun.* **200**, 142–148.

SECTION III

Nitric oxide, bone cell function and osteoporosis

10

Nitric oxide and osteoblast function

FRANCIS J. HUGHES, LEE D. K. BUTTERY, MIKA
V. J. HUKKANEN and JULIA M. POLAK

10.1 Introduction

The osteoblast is the mature differentiated cell responsible for bone formation. The cell is derived from mesenchymal precursor cells that reside in the adjacent tissues and the bone marrow stromal cell populations. Classic experiments on bone cell kinetics demonstrate that osteoblasts are post-mitotic cells with a finite life span and are continually replaced by the proliferation and differentiation of cells from the adjacent progenitor cell populations, although the precise lineage and differentiation stages of the cells are uncertain (Aubin, Turksen and Heersche, 1993). Cells of the osteoblast lineage in culture exhibit a similar repertoire of proliferative and differentiation responses in that proliferating cells in subconfluent cultures do not express osteoblastic features but subsequently show a temporally ordered pattern of expression of osteoblastic genes during differentiation following growth arrest (Stein and Lian, 1993).

During physiological growth and turnover, bone deposition is predictably linked to osteoclastic bone resorption in that a wave of bone resorption is followed by a period of deposition in a process often referred to as coupling. This process permits the turnover of bone (and provides a mechanism of calcium homeostasis) while preserving total bone mass. Perturbations of the coupling process may result in dysregulated bone turnover with increased bone formation and resorption or result in net bone loss following increased bone resorption and decreased bone formation, as is seen in the bone loss associated with chronic inflammatory diseases such as RA, periodontal disease and osteoporosis.

The osteoblast is the pivotal cell involved in cell signalling during the regulation of bone metabolism. Bone formation is controlled by a wide range of endocrine factors such as 1,25-dihydroxy vitamin D_3 and PTH, and by paracrine factors such as many growth factors, cytokines and eicosanoids. In addition, bone resorption is also controlled largely by the interaction of endocrine and paracrine factors with receptors present on the osteoblasts, which then in turn regulate osteoclast function.

Although the nature of these signalling molecules and their actions in bone have been studied extensively, interpretation of some of the data is complicated by the use of a wide range of experimental systems and models for these studies. For

Table 10.1 *Summary of studies of NO production by osteoblasts in vitro*

Reference	Source of osteoblasts	Stimuli	Outcome	Remarks
Lowik *et al.*, 1994	Primary rat calvaria cells: UMR 106 rat osteosarcoma cells; mouse long bone cultures	TNF, IFN, IL-1, LPS	NO_2^- production ↑	Associated with ↓ bone resorption No effect of 1,25-dihydroxy vitamin D_3 Slight ↓ with PTH ↓ with TGFβ
Ralston *et al.*, 1994	Primary human osteoblasts	TNF, IFN, IL-1, LPS	NO_2^- production ↑ RT-PCR for iNOS	Associated with ↑cGMP and ↓ proliferation No effects of 1,25-dihydroxy vitamin D_3 and PTH
Damoulis and Hauschka, 1994	MC3T3 E1 mouse cell line	TNF, IFN, IL-1, LPS	NO_2^- production ↑ Citrulline release ↑	
Riancho *et al.*, 1995a	MG-63 human osteosarcoma; ROS 17/2.8 rat osteosarcoma	TNF, IFN, IL-1, LPS, 1,25-dihydroxy vitamin D_3	Conversion of ^{14}C-Arg to citrulline ↑ RT-PCR for iNOS and cNOS	Associated with ↑ proliferation, alkaline phosphatase, IL-6 production
Hukkanen *et al.*, 1995	Primary rat calvaria cells; MC3T3 E1 mouse cell line; MG-63 human osteosarcoma; ROS17/2.8 rat osteosarcoma	TNF, IFN, IL-1, LPS	NO_2^- production ↑ RT-PCR, IHC, Western blot for iNOS	Associated with ↓ proliferation, alkaline phosphatase, osteocalcin LPS ↓ IFN-induced NO
Pitsillides *et al.*, 1995	Vertebral and ulnal organ cultures; rat primary long bone osteoblasts; chick osteocytes	Mechanical loading	NO_2^- production ↑ RT-PCR for nNOS and iNOS	
Klein-Nulend *et al.*, 1995	Primary chick osteocytes; primary mouse calvaria cells	Pulsatile fluid flow	NO detection by chemiluminescence ↑	NO inhibitors blocked PGE$_2$ production; effect not seen in periosteal fibroblasts

example, although it is possible to demonstrate the ability of a number of inflammatory cytokines to induce bone resorption, it is not altogether clear which, if any, cytokines are of particular importance in a specific disease process. Furthermore, the relationship between different signalling molecules within the cytokine network is usually complex and probably shows considerable redundancy, with a variety of signalling pathways resulting in a similar outcome on cell function. Some of these issues can now be addressed by powerful techniques such as 'gene knockouts', antisense inhibition of expression of specific factors, and the availability of specific inhibitors for pharmacological control of signalling molecules.

Recent evidence implicates NO as a new potentially important signalling molecule in the regulation of bone metabolism in health and disease. This evidence includes firstly the demonstration of the production of NO and the expression of NOS by osteoblasts, secondly the demonstration of functional modulation of bone cells by NO and, thirdly, the elucidation of some of the potential target molecules for the action of NO in bone metabolism. The available evidence to date is certainly incomplete and much further work is required to discern the true place of this ubiquitous signalling mechanism in the control of bone cell function.

10.2 NO production in osteoblasts

10.2.1 Evidence for the production of NO

NO is produced by the action of NOS enzymes on L-arginine, which results in the formation of NO plus citrulline. NO will further react to form nitrites and nitrates, which are the stable end products of NO metabolism. As discussed in Chapter 1, three main NOS enzyme isoforms have been described; the constitutively expressed eNOS and nNOS and the inducible iNOS. The action of constitutively expressed NOS enzymes is calcium dependent and the enzymes are rapidly activated (within seconds) following exposure to a variety of stimuli such as calcium ionophores and acetylcholine to produce relatively low levels of NO. iNOS expression is induced in a wide range of cell types following exposure to cytokines such as IFN-γ, IL-1 and TNFα or to bacterial LPS. In contrast to the constitutive enzymes, iNOS expression is induced slowly over many hours, is dependent on RNA transcription and *de novo* protein synthesis and results in the production of large amounts of NO.

A number of studies have now described the production of NO and the expression of iNOS following cytokine and LPS stimulation in osteoblasts *in vitro*, These studies have utilized a number of different primary and established osteoblast and osteoblastic osteosarcoma cell lines from human, murine and rat sources but show a consistency of results suggesting a general ability of osteoblasts to express iNOS and to produce NO (Damoulis and Hauschka, 1994; Lowik *et al.*, 1994; Ralston *et al.*, 1994; Hukkanen *et al.*, 1995; Riancho *et al.*, 1995a). A summary of these studies is provided in Table 10.1. In general NO production has been measured by the accumulation of nitrite in medium using the Griess reagent, which although specific for nitrite is a relatively insensitive assay (Green *et al.*, 1982). Using this method, small levels of nitrite accumulation are seen following stimulation with single cytokines including IFN-γ, IL-1 and TNFα and with LPS. However, combinations of cytokines, particularly those which include IFN-γ, show strong synergistic actions, with final nitrite concentrations reaching up to 100 μM in some experiments. Nitrite production is dose and time dependent, with accumulation initially seen after 12–24 h and a maximum reached after 48 h of treatment. That nitrite accumulation is genuinely the result of NO production is confirmed by the findings that the effect can be blocked with L-arginine analogues such as L-NMMA, L-NNA and L-NAME, all of which are competitive inhibitors of NOS enzymes. Taken together, the data also suggest that osteotrophic hormones such as PTH and 1,25-dihydroxy vitamin D_3 do not stimulate NO production, although contrary evidence does exist, at least with 1,25-dihydroxy vitamin D_3 (Riancho *et al.*, 1995b).

The studies to date have demonstrated the ability of all the osteoblastic cell lines tested to produce NO, but there are notable variations in the amount of NO produced in different cell lines and in different studies. Although caution needs to be exercised in comparing data from different studies, the amount of NO produced utilizing osteosarcoma-derived cell lines is markedly less than that from primary rat and human osteoblasts and the MC3T3 clonally derived murine osteoblastic line. It is not clear if this observation has significance to the situation *in vivo*, but it is tempting to speculate that NO production may vary between cells at different differentiation stages of the osteoblast lineage.

10.2.2 Expression of NOS enzymes

In the above studies, the role of the iNOS enzyme has been demonstrated by showing induction of gene expression by RT-PCR and Northern blotting (Ralston *et al.* 1994; Hukkanen *et al.*, 1995; Riancho *et al.*, 1995a,b), expression of iNOS protein by immunocytochemistry and Western blotting (Hukkanen *et al.*, 1995), and enzyme activity by demonstration of the conversion of [^{14}C]-arginine to citrulline (Riancho *et al.*, 1995a). The iNOS enzyme is further implicated by the dependence of NO production on new RNA and protein synthesis, absence of calcium dependence (using chelating agents such as ethylene guanidine tetraacetic acid (EGTA)) and the partial inhibition of NO production by dexamethasone.

In addition to the clear demonstration of NO production by induction of iNOS by cytokines, there is now some evidence for the expression of the constitutive endothelial and neuronal forms of NOS in osteoblasts and in osteocytes, and its regulation by mechanical stimuli such as loading and pulsatile fluid flow (Chapters 11, 14–16; Klein-Nulend *et al.*, 1995; Pitsillides *et al.*, 1995; Riancho *et al.*, 1995a). In these studies, mechanical stimuli resulted in rapid release of low concentrations of NO within a few minutes of stimulation, which suggests a further role for NO in mediating the effects of mechanical stimuli on bone metabolism.

Although all of these studies demonstrate the ability of osteoblasts to produce

NO *in vitro*, in fact there are few definitve data that show the production *in vivo*. However, studies have demonstrated increased NO production and the expression of iNOS in inflammatory arthritides, providing some evidence for their potential importance in disease pathogenesis (Farrell *et al.*, 1992; Cannon *et al.*, 1996; Grabowski *et al.*, 1996a; Grabowski, Macpherson and Ralston, 1996b; Ueki *et al.*, 1996).

10.3 Effects of NO on osteoblast metabolism

In addition to the production of NO by osteoblasts themselves, as discussed above, chondrocytes, endothelial cells, neurones, osteoclasts and macrophages are all able to release NO within the bone environment and have the potential to modulate osteoblast metabolism by this route. Although there is evidence of the modulation of osteoblast function from studies *in vitro*, the data are somewhat conflicting and the precise importance of these actions remain to be determined.

10.3.1 Osteoblast growth and differentiation

In order to investigate the potential action of NO in regulating osteoblast function, studies either have utilized cytokine-induced NO production in the presence or absence of NOS inhibitors such as L-NMMA or L-NAME or have directly added NO donor molecules such as sodium nitroprusside or 3-morpholinosyndonimine (SIN-1) to osteoblast cultures. In terms of cell proliferation, a combination of IFN-γ, IL-1 and TNFα inhibited both cell proliferation and DNA synthesis in primary human osteoblasts and the osteoblastic cell lines MC3T3-E1, MG-63 and ROS17/2.8 (Ralston *et al.*, 1994; Hukkanen *et al.*, 1995); this effect was reversed using L-NMMA or L-NAME, suggesting the activity was dependent on NO production. In complete contrast to these findings, studies by Riancho and co-workers demonstrated stimulation of cell proliferation is osteosarcoma cell lines by cytokine-induced NO (Riancho *et al.*, 1995b). This study also demonstrated that NO may play a role in production of IL-6 in the human osteosarcoma line MG-63.

Similar discrepancies are also seen among different studies of the expression of markers of osteoblast differentiation, with evidence for NO reducing expression of alkaline phosphatase and osteocalcin in some studies (Ralston *et al.*, 1994; Hukkanen *et al.*, 1995), while in others stimulation of alkaline phosphatase activity has been reported (Riancho *et al.*, 1995b). On the face of it, these contradictory results are difficult to reconcile, and further studies would be useful to try to clarify the situation. However, the variations may be the result of factors such as the cell lines studied, culture conditions utilized in the different studies or differences in the differentiation status of the cultures. Primary osteoblast cultures are heterogenous populations with osteoblastic cells at both early and later stages of differentiation, and even a clonally derived cell line may show a degree of heterogeneity of differentiation stage according to the cell density and proliferative status of the culture (Hughes and Aubin, 1997). It is clear that osteoblastic cells may show distinct responses to external stimuli according to their differentiation stage; indeed, the literature contains a number of apparently contradictory studies describing both inhibitory and stimulatory responses of osteoblastic cells to cytokines, most notably following stimulation with IL-1 (Stashenko *et al.*, 1987; Ikeda *et al.*, 1988; Ohmori *et al.*, 1988; Ellies and Aubin, 1990; Evans, Bunning and Russell, 1990; Taichman and Hauschka, 1992).

In addition to these explanations for the variations in results in different studies, it is also possible that the data are the result of bi-phasic effects of NO on osteoblastic activity, with low concentrations being stimulatory and high concentrations inhibitory. Such a bi-phasic effect has been suggested regarding the regulation of osteoclastic bone resorption by NO (Brandi *et al.*, 1995; Ralston and Grabowski, 1996). Despite the ultimate uncertainty about the functional significance of NO in the control of osteoblast proliferation and metabolism, the data clearly suggest that at least part of the effect of these cytokines on osteoblast function is mediated by NO production.

10.3.2 NO and cytotoxicity

A further potential confounding variable in the above studies, and a potentially important pathogenic mechanism in inflammatory bone disease, is the possible cytotoxic effects of NO. NO may react with superoxide to form highly reactive species such as peroxynitrite, which may induce apoptotic or necrotic cell death (Szabo, 1996). In addition, there is evidence that NO itself may induce apoptotic cell death in a variety of cell types including thymocytes, macrophages and chondrocytes (Blanco *et al.*, 1995; Brune, Mohr and Messmer, 1996; Fehsel, Kroncke and Kolb-Bachofen, 1996; Okuda *et al.*, 1996). We have recently found that cytokine-induced NO or exogenous NO donors can induce apoptotic cell death in cultured osteoblasts, as demonstrated by induction of DNA strand breaks, characteristic ultrastructural changes and increased cytotoxicity (Hughes *et al.*, 1995 and unpublished data).

Overall, it is clear that NO may have an important role in mediating the effects of inflammatory cytokines on osteoblast metabolism. However, as yet there is relatively little information as to the potential role of lower concentrations of NO, such as may be seen physiologically, in regulating bone cells.

10.4 Potential molecular targets for the action of NO in osteoblasts

The mechanism of signal transduction of NO involves its reaction with iron-containing enzymes, resulting in conformational changes of the protein and enzyme activation. Potential target enzymes for NO have been identified, which include guanylyl cyclase and COX. Other potential target enzymes include the proliferation-associated enzyme ribonucleotide reductase (Lepoivre *et al.*, 1990), but no doubt there are many more potential targets that remain to be elucidated.

10.4.1 Guanylyl cyclase

Guanylyl cyclase is the classical molecular target for NO. Its activity causes rapid elevation of cGMP and is responsible for many of the physiological activities of NO, such as endothelium-derived relaxing activity (Moncada *et al.*, 1991). While NO has been shown to produce rapid elevation of cGMP in osteoblasts exposed to NO, there is little information about the possible importance of this signalling pathway in mediating NO-induced modulation of osteoblast function; indeed, there is evidence that cGMP production is not required for the functional modulation of osteoclasts by NO (MacIntyre *et al.*, 1991; Ralston *et al.*, 1994; Ralston and Grabowski, 1996).

There is a surprising paucity of information regarding the role of the cGMP signalling pathway in the modulation of osteoblast function. Previous studies have demonstrated the localization of cGMP within osteoblasts and the induction of guanylyl cyclase by stimulation with C-natriuretic peptide and mechanical loading (Rodan *et al.*, 1975; Davidovitch, Montgomery and Shanfeld, 1977; Davidovitch *et al.*, 1978; Fukushima and Gay, 1991; Inoue *et al.*, 1996; Suda *et al.*, 1996). This last observation may be of particular interest given the recent demonstration of NO production by osteoblasts in response to mechanical loading (Chapters 14–16). A couple of studies of the effects of cGMP on bone cells have been reported where cells have been treated with the stable analogue 8-bromo-cyclic GMP or with C-natriuretic peptide and these suggest a possible role for cGMP in increasing osteoblast differentiation. 8-Bromo-cyclic GMP has been shown to increase the formation of bone nodules and to increase expression of the differentiated osteoblast markers alkaline phosphatase and osteocalcin (Inoue *et al.*, 1995) in rat calvaria cell cultures. C-natriuretic peptide and 8-bromo-cyclic GMP treatment also increased expression of osteoblastic markers and decreased proliferation in the MC3T3-E1 murine osteoblastic cell line. Clearly, given the relatively few studies that have addressed this issue, attempts to interpret these data as a general effect of cGMP in bone cells should be treated with considerable caution.

10.4.2 Prostaglandins

The action of COX is the rate-limiting step for the production of prostaglandins from arachidonic acid following its release from cell membranes by the action of the enzyme phospholipase A_2. Prostaglandins have profound but complex effects on bone metabolism, including stimulation of osteoclastic bone resorption and a bi-phasic effect on osteoblastic cells: prostaglandins are mitogenic at low concentrations but may be inhibitory at higher concentrations (Raisz, Pilbeam and Fall, 1993). As COX enzymes contain a haem group at their centre, they are potential target enzymes for the action of NO, and studies have demonstrated the ability of NO to activate COX and increase prostaglandin production in a number of cell types (Chapter 7; Franchi *et al.*, 1994; Davidge *et al.*, 1995; Salvemini *et al.*,

1993, 1994, 1995). In addition to these effects on COX-2 activation, we have recently found that NO can also stimulate COX-2 mRNA and protein expression in cultured osteoblasts by both transcriptional and post-transcriptional mechanisms, and that cytokine-induced prostaglandin production is regulated by both NO-dependent and NO-independent pathways (Buttery *et al.*, 1995; F. J. Hughes, L. Buttery, M. Hukkanen, A. O'Donnell, J. MacLouf and J. M. Polak, unpublished data). In support of a possible relationship between NO and prostaglandin production, the induction of PGE_2 production in osteoblasts by pulsatile fluid flow has recently been shown to be blocked by the NOS inhibitor L-NNA (Klein-Nulend *et al.*, 1995). In contrast to these studies, the NO donor *S*-nitroso-*N*-acetylpenicillamine (SNAP) failed to stimulate PGE_2 production by mouse calvaria organ cultures, and there is little evidence as yet to demonstrate that the effects of NO on bone metabolism are prostaglandin dependent (Ralston and Grabowski, 1996). Again the possibility exists of bi-phasic effects of NO, in which the actions of low concentrations of NO are mediated by factors such as cGMP and prostaglandins, but at higher concentrations its actions are controlled by other mechanisms.

10.5 Conclusions

There is now clear evidence for the production of NO by osteoblasts and the expression of the iNOS enzyme in response to stimulation with cytokines such as IFN-γ, IL-1 and TNFα. In addition, there is increasing evidence for the expression of constitutive forms of the NOS enzyme, which may be regulated physiologically by mechanical forces and possibly other stimuli. The data implicate NO as a potentially important modulator of bone metabolism during inflammatory bone diseases, although the precise role of this molecule in these disease states requires further study. It is also clear that the osteoblast is a potential target cell for the action of NO, although much of the detail of its activities remains to be clarified. Important signal transduction mechanisms may include the guanylyl cyclase pathway and the production of prostaglandins, but it is clear that other mechanisms will also prove to be important. Most of the work to date on the actions of NO in bone metabolism have utilized cytokine stimulation or NO donors, resulting in high concentrations of NO production, as seen in pathological states. It seems highly likely that NO may also have profound effects on osteoblast metabolism at much lower 'physiological' concentrations and that much further work is required to understand clearly the importance of this molecule in bone biology.

Acknowledgements

The authors' studies were supported by Medical Research Council project grant number G9409774MA, the Maurice Wohl Charitable Foundation and the BUPA Medical Foundation.

References

Aubin, J. E., Turksen, K. and Heersche, J. N. M. (1993) Osteoblastic cell lineage. In *Cellular and Molecular Biology of Bone* (ed. M. Noda), pp. 1–45. Academic Press, San Diego.

Blanco, F. J., Ochs, R. L., Schwarz, H. and Lotz, M. (1995) Chondrocyte apoptosis induced by nitric oxide. *Am. J. Pathol.* **146**, 75–85.

Brandi, M. L., Hukkanen, M., Umeda, T. *et al.*, (1995) Bidirectional regulation of osteoclast function by nitric oxide synthase isoforms. *Proc. Natl. Acad. Sci. USA* **92**, 2954–2958.

Brune, B., Mohr, S. and Messmer, U. K. (1996) Protein thiol modification and apoptotic cell death as cGMP-independent nitric oxide (NO) signaling pathways. *Rev. Physio. Biochem. Pharmacol.* **127**, 1–30.

Buttery, L. D. K., Hukkanen, M., O'Donnell, A., Polak, J. and Hughes, F. J. (1995) Nitric oxide dependent and independent induction of prostaglandin synthesis in osteoblasts (Abstract 11). *Bone* **17**, 560.

Cannon, G. W., Openshaw, S. J., Hibbs, J. B. Jr, Hoidal, J. R., Huecksteadt, T. P. and Griffiths, M. M. (1996) Nitric oxide production during adjuvant-induced and collagen-induced arthritis. *Arthritis Rheum.* **39**, 1677–1684.

Damoulis, P. D. and Hauschka, P. V. (1994) Cytokines induce nitric oxide production in mouse osteoblasts. *Biochem. Biophys. Res. Commun.* **201**, 924–931.

Davidge, S. T., Baker, P. N., Laughlin, M. K. and Roberts, J. M. (1995) Nitric oxide produced by endothelial cells increases production of eicosanoids through activation of prostaglandin H synthase. *Circ. Res.* **77**, 274–283.

Davidovitch, Z., Montgomery, P. C. and Shanfeld, J. L. (1977) Cellular localization and concentration of bone cyclic nucleotides in response to acute PTE administration. *Calcif. Tiss. Res.* **24**, 81–91.

Davidovitch, Z., Montgomery, P. C., Yost, R. W. and Shanfeld, J. L. (1978) Immunohistochemical localization of cyclic nucleotides in mineralized tissues: mechanically-stressed osteoblasts *in vivo. Anat. Rec.* **192**, 363–373.

Ellies, L. G. and Aubin, J. E. (1990) Temporal sequence of interleukin 1 alpha-mediated stimulation and inhibition of bone formation by isolated fetal rat calvaria cells *in vitro. Cytokine* **2**, 430–437.

Evans, D. B., Bunning, R. A. and Russell, R. G. (1990) The effects of recombinant human interleukin-1 beta on cellular proliferation and the production of prostaglandin E_2, plasminogen activator, osteocalcin and alkaline phosphatase by osteoblast-like cells derived from human bone. *Biochem. Biophys. Res. Commun.* **166**, 208–216.

Farrell, A. J., Blake, D. R., Palmer, R. M. and Moncada, S. (1992) Increased concentrations of nitrite in synovial fluid and serum samples suggest increased nitric oxide synthesis in rheumatic diseases. *Ann. Rheum. Dis.* **51**, 1219–1222.

Fehsel, K., Kroncke, K. D. and Kolb-Bachofen, V. (1996) NO as a physiological signal molecule that triggers thymocyte apoptosis. *Adv. Exp. Med. Biol.* **387**, 195–198.

Franchi, A. M., Chaud, M., Rettori, V., Suburo, A., McCann, S. M. and Gimeno, M. (1994) Role of nitric oxide in eicosanoid synthesis and uterine motility in estrogen-treated rat uteri. *Proc. Natl. Acad. Sci., USA* **91**, 539–543.

Fukushima, O. and Gay, C. V. (1991) Ultrastructural localization of guanylate cyclase in bone cells. *J. Histochem. Cytochem.* **39**, 529–535.

Grabowski, P. S., England, A. J., Dykhuizen, R. *et al.* (1996*a*) Elevated nitric oxide production in rheumatoid arthritis. Detection using the fasting urinary nitrate:creatinine ratio. *Arthritis Rheum.* **39**, 643–647.

Grabowski, P. S., Macpherson, H. and Ralston, S. H. (1996*b*) Nitric oxide production in cells derived from the human joint. *Br. J. Rheumatol.* **35**, 207–212.

Green, L. C., Wagner, D. A., Glogowski, J., Skipper, P. L., Wishnok, J. S. and Tannenbaum, S. R. (1982) Analysis of nitrate, nitrite, and [^{15}N] nitrate in bioligical fluids. *Anal. Biochem.* **126**, 131–138.

Hughes, F. J. and Aubin, J. E. (1997) Culture of cells of the osteoblast lineage. In *Methods in Bone Biology* (ed. T. R. Arnett and B. Henderson), in press. London, Chapman & Hall.

Hughes, F. J., Ghazi, R., Hukkanen, M., Buttery, L. and Polak, J. (1995) Cytokine-induced apoptosis in osteoblast cultures mediated by nitric oxide (Abstract 31). *Bone* **17**, 565.

Hukkanen, M., Hughes, F., Buttery, L. *et al.* (1995) Cytokine-stimulated expression of inducible nitric oxide synthase by mouse, rat and human osteoblast-like cell and its functional role in osteoblast metabolic activity. *Endocrinology* **136**, 5445–5453.

Ikeda, E., Kusaka, M., Hakeda, Y., Yokota, K., Kumegawa, M. and Yamamoto, S. (1988) Effect of interleukin 1 beta on osteoblastic clone MC3T3-E1 cells. *Calcif. Tiss. Int.* **43**, 162–166.

Inoue, A., Hiruma, Y., Hirose, S., Yamaguchi, A. and Hagiwara, H. (1995) Reciprocal regulation by cyclic nucleotides of the differentiation of rat osteoblast-like cells and mineralization of nodules. *Biochem. Biophys. Res. Commun.* **215**, 1104–1110.

Inoue, A., Hiruma, Y., Hirose, S. *et al.* (1996) Stimulation by C-type natriuretic peptide of the differentiation of clonal osteoblastic MC3T3-E1 cells. *Biochem. Biophys. Res. Commun.* **221**, 703–707.

Klein-Nulend, J., Semeins, C. M., Ajubi, N. E., Nijweide, P. J. and Burger, E. H. (1995) Pulsating fluid flow increases nitric oxide (NO) synthesis by osteocytes but not periosteal fibroblasts – correlation with prostaglandin upregulation. *Biochem. Biophys. Res. Commun.* **217**, 640–648.

Lepoivre, M., Chenais, B., Yapo, A., Lemaire, G., Thelander, L. and Tenu, J.-P. (1990) Alterations of ribonucleotide reductase activity following induction of the nitrite-generating pathway in adenocarcinoma cells. *J. Biol. Chem.* **165**, 14 143–14 149.

Lowik, C. W., Nibbering, P. H., van de Ruit, M. and Papapoulos, S. E. (1994) Inducible production of nitric oxide in osteoblast-like cells and in fetal mouse bone explants is associated with suppression of osteoclastic bone resorption. *J. Clin. Invest.* **93**, 1465–1472.

MacIntyre, I., Zaidi, M., Alam, A. S. *et al.* (1991) Osteoclastic inhibition: an action of nitric oxide not mediated by cyclic GMP. *Proc. Natl. Acad. Sci., USA* **88**, 2936–2940.

Moncada, S., Palmer, R. M. J., Hibbs, J. R. and Higgs, A. E. (1991) Nitric oxide: physiology, pathophysiology and pharmacology. *Pharmacol. Rev.* **43**, 109–118.

Ohmori, Y., Hanazawa, S., Amano, S., Hirose, K., Kumegawa, M. and Kitano, S. (1988) Effects of recombinant human interleukin 1 alpha and interleukin 1 beta on cell growth and alkaline phosphatase of the mouse osteoblastic cell line MC3T3-E1. *Biochim. Biophys. Acta* **970**, 22–30.

Okuda, Y., Sakoda, S., Shimaoka, M. and Yanagihara, T. (1996) Nitric oxide induces apoptosis in mouse splenic T lymphocytes. *Immunol. Lett.* **52**, 135–138.

Pitsillides, A. A., Rawlinson, S. C., Suswillo, R. F., Bourrin, S., Zaman, G. and Lanyon, L. E. (1995) Mechanical strain-induced NO production by bone cells: a possible role in adaptive bone (re)modeling? *FASEB J.* **9**, 1614–1622.

Raisz, L. G., Pilbeam, C. C. and Fall, P. M. (1993) Prostaglandins: mechanisms of action and regulation of production in bone. *Osteoporosis Int.* **3**(Suppl. 1), S136–S140.

Ralston, R. H. and Grabowski, P. S. (1996) Mechanisms of cytokine induced bone resorption: role of nitric oxide, cyclic guanosine monophosphate and prostaglandins. *Bone* **19**, 29–33.

Ralston, S. H., Todd, D., Helfrich, M., Benjamin, N. and Grabowski, P. S. (1994) Human osteoblast-like cells produce nitric oxide and express inducible nitric oxide synthase. *Endocrinology* **135**, 330–336.

Riancho, J. A., Salas, E., Zarrabeitia, M. T. *et al.* (1995*a*) Expression and functional role of nitric oxide synthase in osteoblast-like cells. *J. Bone Min. Res* **10**, 439–446.

Riancho, J. A., Zarrabeitia, M. T.. Fernandez-Luna, J. L. and Gonzalez-Macias, J. (1995*b*) Mechanisms controlling nitric oxide synthesis in osteoblasts. *Mol. Cell. Endocrinol.* **107**, 87–92.

Rodan, G. A., Bourret, L. A., Harvey, A. and Mensi, T. (1975) Cyclic AMP and cyclic GMP: mediators of the mechanical effects on bone remodelling. *Science* **189**, 467–469.

Salvemini, D., Misko, T. P., Masferrer, J. L. Seibert, K., Currie, M. G. and Needleman, P. (1993) Nitric oxide activates cyclooxygenase enzymes. *Proc. Natl. Acad. Sci., USA* **90**, 7240–7244.

Salvemini, D., Seibert, K., Masferrer, J. L., Misko, T. P., Currie, M. G. and Needleman, P. (1994) Endogenous nitric oxide enhances prostaglandin production in a model of renal inflammation. *J. Clin. Invest.* **93**, 1940–1947.

Salvemini, D., Manning, P. T., Zweifel, B. S. *et al.* (1995) Dual inhibition of nitric oxide and prostaglandin production contributes to the antiinflammatory properties of nitric oxide synthase inhibitors. *J. Clin. Invest.* **96** 301–308.

Stashenko, P., Dewhirst, F. E., Rooney, M. L., Desjardins, L. A. and Heeley, J. D. (1987) Interleukin-1 beta is a potent inhibitor of bone formation *in vitro*. *J. Bone Min. Res.* **2**, 559–565.

Stein, G. S. and Lian, J. B. (1993) Molecular mechanisms mediating proliferation/differentiation interrelationships during progressive development of the osteoblast phenotype. *Endocrine Rev.* **14**, 424–442.

Suda, M., Tanaka, K., Fukushima, M. *et al.* (1996) C-type natriuretic peptide as an autocrine/paracrine regulator of osteoblast. Evidence for possible presence of bone natriuretic peptide system. *Biochem. Biophys. Res. Commun.* **223**, 1–6.

Szabo, C. (1996) DNA strand breakage and activation of poly-ADP ribosyltransferase: a cytotoxic pathway triggered by peroxynitrite. *Free Radical Biol. Med.* **21**, 855–869.

Taichman, R. S. and Hauschka, P. V. (1992) Effects of interleukin-1 beta and tumor necrosis factor-alpha on osteoblastic expression of osteocalcin and mineralized extracellular matrix *in vitro*. *Inflammation* **16**, 587–601.

Ueki, Y., Miyake, S., Tominaga, Y. and Eguchi, K. (1996) Increased nitric oxide levels in patients with rheumatoid arthritis. *J. Rheumatol.* **23**, 230–236.

11

Nitric oxide as a mediator of cytokine effects on bone

STUART H. RALSTON

11.1 Introduction

NO was first discovered to be a mediator of smooth muscle relaxation and since has emerged as a pleiotropic mediator with effects on several tissues and organ systems. While initial work focused on the effects of NO on the vascular and nervous systems, an accumulating body of evidence has now emerged to suggest that NO also plays a key role as a mediator of cellular activity in bone. This chapter reviews the factors that regulate synthesis of NO in bone-derived cells, the isoforms of NOS expressed in bone, the biological effects of NO on bone cell function and the effects of NO donors and inhibitors on bone *in vivo*, with particular reference to the role of NO as a mediator of cytokine actions on bone and bone-derived cells.

11.2 Expression of NOS isoforms in bone and bone-derived cells

Immunohistochemical studies of whole bone and cultured bone-derived cells have shown evidence of widespread eNOS expression in bone marrow stromal cells, osteoblasts, osteocytes and osteoclasts (Brandi *et al.*, 1995; Chow, Chambers and Fox, 1996; Helfrich *et al.*, 1997). While nNOS mRNA has also been detected in whole bone and bone marrow cultures by RT-PCR (Pitsillides *et al.*, 1995b; Helfrich *et al.*, 1997), this isoform has proved more difficult to detect in bone and cultured bone-derived cells by immunohistochemical techniques. We have not detected expression of nNOS in cultured bone-derived cells for example, and others have also failed to detect evidence of nNOS in whole bone using immunohisto-chemical techniques (Schmidt *et al.*, 1992).

Although low levels of iNOS transcripts have been detected in whole bone and cultured osteoblasts by RT-PCR, we have found no evidence of iNOS protein by immunostaining in bone sections or in cultured osteoblasts under basal conditions. We have, however, detected iNOS expression in short-term cultures of bone marrow macrophages even in the absence of cytokine stimulation, suggesting that these cells may 'constitutively' express iNOS at least *in vitro* (Helfrich *et al.*, 1997).

11.3 Regulation of NOS expression in bone

Most bone cells can be induced to produced iNOS in response to stimulation with cytokines and/or endotoxin (Lowik *et al.*, 1994; Ralston *et al.*, 1994, 1995; van't Hof and Ralston, 1995; Ralston and Grabowski, 1996). In general, combinations of cytokines are better stimulators of NO production in bone cells than single cytokines; in turn, rodent cells are more responsive to the stimulatory effects of single cytokines than human cells (MacPherson *et al.*, 1995). Calciotrophic hormones such as PTH and 1,25-dihydroxy vitamin D_3, in contrast, do not appear to stimulate NO production (Ralston *et al.*, 1994, 1995); in one study, 1,25-dihydroxy vitamin D_3 inhibited cytokine-induced NO production by rodent osteoblasts (Lowik *et al.*, 1994). Published data on cytokine-induced iNOS expression by mature osteoclasts are controversial; our own studies in bone marrow co-cultures have shown that the majority of cytokine-induced NO derives from osteoblasts (van't Hof and Ralston, 1996) and we recently have failed to detect iNOS protein or mRNA in cultured osteoclasts even after cytokine stimulation (Helfrich *et al.*, 1997). Nonetheless, weak iNOS expression has been deteced by others in osteoclasts *in vivo* (Chow *et al.*, 1996) and in pre-osteoclastic cell lines *in vitro* (Brandi *et al.*, 1995).

While osteoblasts in culture produce low or undetectable amounts of NO under basal conditions, as assessed by nitrite measurements in conditioned medium (Ralston *et al.*, 1994), these cells do possess some basal NOS activity, which can be detected using the arginine–citrulline assay (Riancho *et al.*, 1995). It is probable that eNOS accounts for much of this activity, since it is inhibited by EGTA (Riancho *et al.*, 1995) and since osteoblasts have not been consistently found to express nNOS by RT-PCR or immunohistochemical assays (Helfrich *et al.*, 1997). Currently, the function of low level 'constitutive' NOS expression in osteoblasts is unclear, although it has been suggested that it may play a role in osteoblast growth and cytokine production (Riancho *et al.*, 1995).

11.4 Effects of NO on bone cell function

11.4.1 Bone-resorbing cells

The first studies of NO effects on bone cell activity were those of McIntyre and co-workers, who showed that dissolved NO gas and NO-generating agents inhibited cell spreading and bone resorption in rat osteoclast cultures (Chapter 12; MacIntyre *et al.*, 1991). Although these observations were largely of pharmacological interest because of the high NO concentrations used, the subsequent demonstration that bone cells produce NO constitutively and in response to cytokines and mechanical strain (Lowik *et al.*, 1994; Hukkanen *et al.*, 1995; Klein-Nulend *et al.*, 1995; Pitsillides *et al.*, 1995a; Ralston *et al.*, 1995; Riancho *et al.*, 1995; van't Hof and Ralston, 1995; Evans and Ralston, 1996) suggest that production of NO within the bone microenvironment may also be important in normal bone physiology.

The inhibitory effects of high NO concentrations on bone resorption has now been confirmed by several investigators (MacIntyre *et al.*, 1991; Kasten *et al.*, 1994; Lowik *et al.*, 1994; Brandi *et al.*, 1995; Ralston *et al.*, 1995; van't Hof and Ralston, 1995). Recent data indicate that not only does NO have an inhibitory effect on mature osteoclasts (MacIntyre *et al.*, 1991; Kasten *et al.*, 1994; Brandi *et al.*, 1995) but also that it inhibits osteoclast formation by inducing apoptosis of early osteoclast progenitors (van't Hof and Ralston, 1995). While proapoptotic effects of NO are well recognized to occur in many cell types, an interesting facet of NO-induced apoptosis in bone is the relative selectivity for osteoclast progenitors, rather than mature osteoclasts or osteoblasts. This is of interest in illustrating that cell type and stage of differentiation influences susceptibility of cells to NO-induced apoptosis and of clinical relevance in showing that NO donors may have therapeutic potential as selective inhibitors of bone resorption *in vivo* (Wimalawansa *et al.*, 1996).

Although high NO concentrations inhibit bone resorption, there is evidence that lower concentrations may be necessary for normal osteoclast function (Brandi *et al.*, 1995) and indeed may act to enhance osteoclast formation and bone resorption induced by certain cytokines. For example, IL-1 and TNF are potent stimulators of bone resorption that have been shown to increase NO production in organ cultures of bone and in bone marrow cultures (Ralston *et al.*, 1995). In these assay systems, bone resorption induced by IL-1 and TNF is inhibited by NOS inhibitors, suggesting that NO produced by these cytokines acts together with other cytokine-induced mediators such as prostaglandins to potentiate bone resorption (Ralston *et al.*, 1995; Ralston and Grabowski, 1996).

11.4.2 Bone-forming cells

The effects of NO on bone formation and osteoblast function are less well characterized than those on bone resorption. It has been suggested that constitutive production of NO may act as an autocrine stimulator of osteoblast growth and cytokine production since NOS inhibitors have been found to inhibit growth and IL-6 production by osteoblast cell lines in arginine-free culture medium (Riancho *et al.*, 1995). Although the above effects were reversed by the NO donor sodium nitroprusside (Riancho *et al.*, 1995), we have found no effects of NOS inhibitors on osteoblast growth under normal culture conditions (Ralston *et al.*, 1994). In view of these discrepancies, it is currently unclear to what extent 'constitutive' NO production regulates normal osteoblast function. While the effects of cNOS on osteoblast function are controversial, there is little doubt that high concentrations of NO, generated pharmacologically by NO donors or by combinations of proinflammatory cytokines, have potent inhibitory effects on osteoblast growth and differentiation (Ralston *et al.*, 1994; Hukkanen *et al.*, 1995). This observation may be relevant in explaining the inhibitory effects of proinflammatory cytokines on bone formation and in explaining the reduced bone formation that has been detected in conditions associated with cytokines activation and the animal model of inflammation-mediated osteopenia (Minne *et al.*, 1984).

11.4.3 Effects of NO on bone metabolism in vivo

Few investigators have looked at the effects of NO on bone *in vivo*. In one study, Kasten *et al.* found evidence of accelerated bone loss in rats treated with the NOS inhibitor aminoguanidine (Kasten *et al.*, 1994). Although these effects were attributed to NO inhibition, inhibitory effects on other enzyme systems cannot be excluded (Peterson *et al.*, 1992). In a further study of ovariectomized rats, NOS inhibitors were found to abolish the anabolic effects of oestrogen on bone, and NO donors were found to increase bone mass (Wimalawansa *et al.*, 1996). This is persuasive evidence in favour of a direct effect of NO on bone turnover, but significant changes in body weight also occurred, raising the possibility of an indirect mechanism of action such as NO-induced changes in appetite and body weight. These studies illustrate the problems that occur in interpreting the results of long-term studies with NO donors or NO inhibitors *in vivo*.

For the moment, the physiological role of the various NOS isoforms in bone remain unclear, but it is probable that these issues will be partly resolved by studies of bone metabolism in NOS knockout mice.

11.5 Clinical relevance of NO in bone diseases

Studies *in vitro* and in animal models suggest that NO could fulfil several possible roles in the regulation of bone metabolism: as a physiological regulator of normal bone cell function, as a mediator of the effects of mechanical strain on bone and as a mediator of cytokine actions in bone.

NO may play an important role as a mediator of bone and tissue damage in inflammatory conditions associated with cytokine activation such as RA. Recent studies have shown that the inhibitory effects of IL-1 on matrix production by cultured chondrocytes is partly mediated by NO (Hickery *et al.*, 1994), and NO has been shown to activate metalloproteinases in cultured chondrocytes (Stefanovic-Racic *et al.*, 1996). Since there is evidence that low NO concentrations stimulate bone resorption (Ralston *et al.*, 1995; Evans and Ralston 1996), it is possible that a gradient of NO production around the inflamed joint may contribute to the increased periarticular bone loss that is a characteristic feature of RA. The well-established vasodilating effects of NO, coupled with a clear demonstration of iNOS expression in blood vessels in RA synovium (Sakurai *et al.*, 1995), suggest that iNOS activation in the RA joint may also be partly responsible for the increased blood flow associated with joint inflammation, which, again, might be expected to increase local bone loss. A pathogenic role of NO in arthritis is further supported by data from animal models, which show that inhibitors of NOS suppress inflammatory arthritis (McCartney-Francis *et al.*, 1993), and clinical studies, which show that diminution of NO production correlates with improvement in clinical and laboratory measures of disease activity (S. H. Ralston, unpublished data).

The assembled data, therefore, show that NO is a potentially important mediator of bone turnover. The challenge now before us is to define the clinical relevance of

NO in bone physiology in humans under normal and pathological circumstances and to explore the therapeutic potential of NO donors and inhibitors in the treatment of bone diseases.

Acknowledgements

I would like to acknowledge the contribution of the following colleagues to the work presented here: Prof. N. Benjamin, Dr D. Evans, Dr P. Grabowski, Dr M. Helfrich, Dr R. van't Hof, Ms H. McPherson, Ms Grace Taylor and Mr D. Todd. I would also like to acknowledge the Arthritis and Rheumatism Council (UK), Action Research and the Scottish Home and Health Department for grant support.

References

Brandi, M. L., Hukkanen, M., Umeda, T. *et al.* (1995) Bidirectional regulation of osteoclast function by nitric oxide synthase isoforms. *Proc. Natl. Acad. Sci. USA* **92**, 2954–2958.

Chow, J. W. M., Chambers, T. J. and Fox, S. W. (1996) Immunolocalisation of nitric oxide synthase in bone cells. *J. Bone Min. Res.* **11**, S270.

Evans, D. M. and Ralston, S. H. (1996) Nitric oxide and bone. *J. Bone Min. Res.* **11**, 300–305.

Helfrich, M. H., Evans, D. M., Grabowski, P. S., Pollock, J. S., Ohshima, H. and Ralston, S. H. (1997) Expression of nitric oxide synthase isoforms in bone and bone cell cultures. *J. Bone Min. Res.* **12**, 1108–1115.

Hickery, M. S., Palmer, R.M. J., Charles, I. G., Moncada, S. and Bayliss, M. T. (1994) The role of nitric oxide in IL-1 induced inhibition of proteoglycan synthesis in human articular cartilage (Abstract). *Br. J. Rheumatol.* **33** (Suppl 1), 92.

Hukkanen, M., Hughes, F. J., Lee, D. *et al.* (1995) Cytokine stimulated expression of inducible nitric oxide synthase by mouse, rat and human osteoblast-like cells and its functional role in osteoblast metabolic activity. *Endocrinology* **136**, 5445–5453.

Kasten, T. P., Collin-Osdoby, P., Patel, N. *et al.* (1994) Potentiation of osteoclast bone resorbing activity by inhibition of nitric oxide synthase. *Proc. Natl. Acad. Sci. USA* **91**, 3569–3573.

Klein-Nulend, J., Semeins, C. M., Ajubi, N. E., Nijweide, P. J. and Burger, E. H. (1995) Pulsating fluid flow increases nitric oxide (NO) synthesis by osteocytes but not periosteal fibroblasts–correlation with prostaglandin up-regulation. *Biochem. Biophys. Res. Commun.* **217**, 640–648.

Lowik, C. W. G. M., Nibbering, P. H., van der Ruit, M. and Papapoulos, S. E. (1994) Inducible production of nitric oxide in osteoblast like cells and in fetal bone explants is associated with supression of osteoclastic bone resorption. *J. Clin. Invest.* **93**, 1465–1472.

MacIntyre, I., Zaid, M., Towhidul Alam, A. S. M. *et al.* (1991). Osteoclast inhibition: an action of nitric oxide not mediated by cyclic GMP. *Proc. Natl. Acad. Sci. USA* **88**, 2936–2940.

MacPherson, H., Noble, B. S. and Ralston, S. H. (1995) Nitric oxide production by human osteoblast-like cells and osteosarcoma cell lines (Abstract). *Calcif. Tiss. Int.* **56**, 431.

McCartney-Francis, N., Allen, J. B., Mizel, D. E. *et al.* (1993) Supression of arthritis by an inhibitor of nitric oxide synthase. *J. Exp. Med.* **178**, 749–754.

Minne, H. W., Pfeilschifter, J., Scharla, S. *et al.* (1984) Inflammation mediated osteopaenia in the rat: a new animal model for pathological loss of bone mass. *Endocrinology* **115**, 50–54.

Peterson, D. A., Peterson, D. C., Archer, S. and Weir, E. K. (1992) The non-specificity of specific nitric oxide synthase inhibitors. *Biochem. Biophys. Res. Commun.* **187**, 797–801.

Pitsillides, A., Rawlinson, S. C. F., Suswillo, R. F. L., Zaman, G., Nijweide, P. J. and Lanyon, L. E. (1995a) Mechanical strain-induced nitric oxide production by osteoblasts and osteocytes. *J. Bone Min. Res.* **10**(suppl. 1), S217.

Pitsillides, A. A., Rawlinson, S. C. F., Suswillo, R. F. L., Bourrin, S., Zaman, G. and Lanyon, L. E. (1995b) Mechanical strain-induced NO production by bone cells: a possible role in adaptive bone (re)modelling? *FASEB J.* **9**, 1614–1622.

Ralston, S. H. and Grabowski, P. S. (1996) Mechanisms of cytokine induced bone resorption: role of nitric oxide, cyclic guanosine monophosphate and prostaglandins. *Bone* **19**, 29–33.

Ralston, S. H., Todd, D., Helfrich, M. H., Benjamin, N. and Grabowski, P. (1994) Human osteoblast-like cells produce nitric oxide and express inducible nitric oxide synthase. *Endocrinology* **135**, 330–336.

Ralston, S.H., Ho, L. P., Helfrich, M. H., Grabowski, P. S., Johnston, P. W. and Benjamin, N. (1995) Nitric oxide: a cytokine-induced regulator of bone resorption. *J. Bone Min. Res.* **10**, 1040–1049.

Riancho, J. A., Salas, E., Zarrabeitia, M. T. *et al.* (1995) Expression and functional role of nitric oxide synthase in osteoblast-like cells. *J. Bone Min. Res.* **10**, 439–446.

Sakurai, H., Koshaka, H., Lui, M. *et al.* (1995) Nitric oxide production and inducible nitric oxide synthase expression in inflammatory arthritides. *J. Clin. Invest.* **96**, 2357–2363.

Schmidt, H. H. W., Gagne, G. D., Nakane, M., Pollock, J. S., Miller, M. F. and Murad, F. (1992). Mapping of neural nitric oxide synthase in the rat suggests frequent co-localisation with NADPH diphorase but not with soluble guanylate cyclase and novel paraneural functions for signal transduction. *J. Histochem. Cytochem.* **40**, 1439–1456.

Stefanovic-Racic, M., Morales, T. I., Taskiran, D., McIntyre, L. A. and Evans, C. H. (1996) The role of nitric oxide in proteoglycan turnover by bovine articular cartilage organ cultures. *J. Immunol.* **156**, 1213–1220.

van't Hof, R. J. and Ralston, S. H. (1995) Cytokine induced nitric oxide production inhibits bone resorption in mouse bone marrow cultures by inducing apoptosis in osteoclast progenitors (Abstract). *Bone* **17**, 587.

van't Hof, R. J. and Ralston, S. H. (1996) Cytokine induced bone resorption in mouse osteoclast cultures: differences between IL-1 and TNF (Absract). *Bone* **17**, 815.

Wimalawansa, S. J., De Marco, G., Gangula, P., Yallampalli, C. (1996) Nitric oxide donor alleviates ovariectomy induced bone loss. *Bone* **18**, 301–304.

12

The osteoclast, bone homeostasis and postmenopausal osteoporosis

LUCIA MANCINI, NILOUFAR MORADI-BIDHENDI and
IAIN MACINTYRE

12.1 Introduction

In this chapter, we shall outline key phases of osteoclast function and show how NO exerts a dominant controlling inhibition of bone resorption by its effect on the osteoclast. Since osteoclast activity produces the bone loss that follows the menopause or is associated with metastatic deposits or arthritis, effective therapeutic prevention of bone loss depends on a thorough understanding of osteoclast function and its physiological modulation.

12.2 Osteoclast activity is a cyclic phenomenon

Osteoclastic resorption occurs in several sequential phases. Firstly, the osteoclast is recruited from marrow stem cells before dividing to produce the active population; control of this replication is probably the most important means of regulating bone resorption. Despite this we still do not fully understand the factors that exert the major effect on the size of the osteoclast population. Mononuclear osteoclasts fuse to produce the multinucleated mature resorbing cell, which then attaches to the bone surface. After attachment, the osteoclast 'spreads', thus increasing in area; subsequent to this spreading, the cell secretes hydrochloric acid followed shortly after by potent proteases. The excavated pit under the cell rapidly fills with acidic fluid containing an increasing concentration of calcium. This dissolution of mineral is dependent on the presence of acid phosphatase, and the mineral removal precedes the proteolytic removal of the underlying collagen framework of the bone. When calcium in the vacuole reaches a certain level, the ion triggers an increase in osteoclast intracellular calcium, which activates the constitutive eNOS within the cell. The gas radical produced in increased amounts by this process produces osteoclast detachment, movement to a fresh site, reattachment and repetition of the whole process. The osteoclast is a highly motile cell, and during its normal resorptive activity it tracks a serpiginous path (Figure 12.1) over the bone surface until a final detachment is followed by apoptosis and cell death. The various stages of the cycle are shown in Figure 12.2.

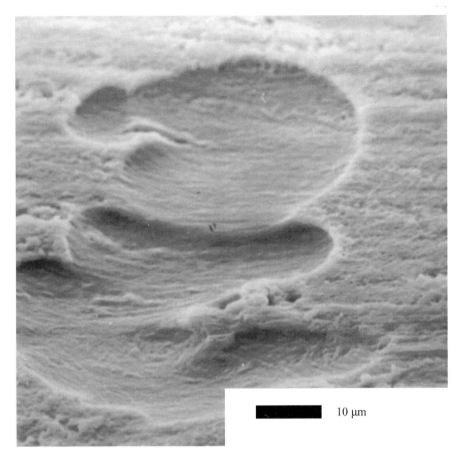

10 μm

Figure 12.1. Scanning electron micrograph of a typical osteoclastic excavation on a bovine cortical bone slice after removal of cells.

12.3 Functions of NO in the osteoclast cycle

NO exerts a powerful inhibitory influence over several of the phases of the osteoclast cycle. NO limits the total osteoclast population by triggering terminal maturation, and by accelerating osteoclast detachment it shortens the resorptive phase (Brandi *et al.*, 1995). Crucially, NO inhibits acid secretion (van Epps-Fung *et al.*, 1994) but it also diminishes the activity of acid phosphatase (L. Mancini, N. Moradi-Bidhendi and I. MacIntyre, unpublished data), perhaps by interaction with the iron atoms in the molecule. The importance of acid phosphatase for bone resorption has been shown by Hayman and Cox (1994) and Zaidi *et al.* (1989). The effects are summarized in Figure 12.3. Most of these actions have been demonstrated *in vitro* and confirmed *in vivo*, although more extensive studies are required before these conclusions can be regarded as established. It is also unclear how these effects of NO interact with the actions of the major osteoclast-regulating hormones, calcitonin and oestradiol. However, it seems likely that an increase in intracellular calcium follows the interaction of calcitonin and oestradiol with the osteoclast cell

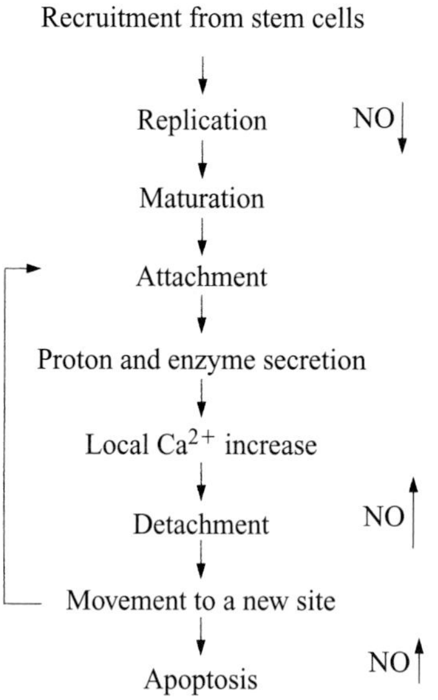

Recruitment from stem cells
Replication
NO
Maturation
Attachment
Proton and enzyme secretion
Local Ca2+ increase
Detachment
NO
Movement to a new site
Apoptosis
NO

Figure 12.2. The osteoclast cycle.

Osteoclast
eNOS
O2−
H2O2
OC detachment
Peroxynitrite
NO
G cyclase
cGMP
OC
replication
Acid
phosphatase
(Fe)
G kinase
?+
+
+
CT
Ca2+
E2
Apoptosis ?
Proton pump
Resorption
H+

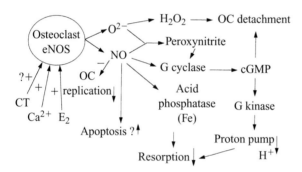

Figure 12.3. eNOS in bone resorption.

membrane receptors for these two hormones. The increased level of intracellular calcium that has been securely documented in the osteoclast-like FLG 29.1 cell (Fiorelli *et al.*, 1996), while exposure of primary neonatal rat osteoclasts to oestradiol (10^{-5} to 10^{-6} M) is followed by the type of cell contraction seen after exposure to calcium or NO. If this still speculative view becomes established, it will identify NO as a major second messenger of the osteoclast-regulating hormones.

12.4 Functions of NO *in vivo*

Certainly the *in vivo* experiments of Kasten *et al.* (1994) and of Wimalawansa *et al.* (1996) are consistent with NO acting as a second messenger as described above. Kasten showed that inhibition of NO production *in vivo* in rats was followed by marked bone loss within a few weeks of administration of the inhibitor. Similarly,

Wimalawansa and colleagues found that inhibition of NOS activity in experimental rats produced very similar changes in bone mass to those seen after oophorectomy. Further, they showed that the effects of oophorectomy were limited or even prevented by administration of NO donors such as nitroglycerine. These findings urgently need confirmation because they could imply that an important part of the effects of oestrogen lack may be deficient production of NO. The specificity of Wimalawansa's findings, however, may be open to question, and experiments in other species are urgently needed. These experimental observations suggest that novel therapeutic agents based on the action of NO in bone may be possible. These might provide an additional weapon to minimize the bone loss after the menopause, in metastatic bone loss or in arthritis.

References

Brandi, M. L., Hukkanen, M., Umeda, T. *et al.* (1995) Bidirectional regulation of osteoclast function by nitric oxide synthase isoforms. *Proc. Natl. Acad. Sci. USA* **92**, 2954–2958.

Fiorelli, G., Gori, F., Frediani, U. *et al.* (1996) Membrane binding sites and nongenomic effects of estrogen in cultured human pre-osteoclastic cells. *J. Steroid Biochem. Mol. Biol.* **59**, 233–240.

Hayman, A. R. and Cox, T. M. (1994) Purple acid phosphatase of the human macrophage and osteoclast *J. Biol. Chem.* **269**, 1294–1300.

Kasten, T. P., Collin-Osdoby, P., Patel, N. *et al.* (1994) Potentiation of osteoclast bone-resorption activity by inhibition of nitric oxide synthase. *Proc. Natl. Acad. Sci. USA* **91**, 3569–3573.

van Epps-Fung, C., Williams, J. P., Cornwell, T. L. *et al.* (1994) Regulation of osteoclastic acid secretion by cGMP-dependent protein kinase. *Biochem. Biophys. Res. Commun.* **204**, 565–571.

Wimalawansa, S. J., De Marco, G., Gangula, P. and Yallampalli, C. (1996) Nitric oxide donor alleviates ovariectomy-induced bone loss. *Bone* **18**, 301–304.

Zaidi, M., Moonga, B., Moss, D. W. and MacIntyre, I. (1989) Inhibition of osteoclastic acid phosphatase abolishes bone resorption. *Biochem. Biophys. Res. Commun.* **159**, 68–71.

Nitric oxide and mechanical factors

13

Modulation of bone blood flow by nitric oxide

IAN D. MCCARTHY

13.1 Introduction

There is increasing interest in the role of the microcirculation in several aspects of bone physiology and patho-physiology. Vascularization precedes osteogenesis, and this observation prompted the suggestion that vessels play an important role in osteogenesis (Trueta, 1963). More and more experimental evidence is now being obtained to support this hypothesis. There is evidence that bone vasculature can modify bone formation through changes in intraosseous pressure (Kelly and Bronk, 1990) and that endothelial cells release factors that modulated osteoclast and osteoblast function (Collin-Osdoby, 1994).

13.2 NO in local control of bone blood flow

13.2.1 Anatomy of the vasculature in bone

Knowledge of the anatomical arrangement of the vessels in the skeleton comes from detailed studies using techniques of vascular casting (Brookes, 1971; Crock, 1996).

The main supply of the long bones is via the nutrient artery. The artery traverses the cortex at an acute angle and does not send off any branches on its route. In the medullary cavity, the nutrient artery divides into ascending and descending medullary branches, and further vessels radiate from these medullary arteries out to the cortex. Therefore, in normal bone, blood flow is principally centrifugal. Exchange vessels within the Haversian canals run in parallel to the long axis of the bone, and it is these vessels that drain into the venules on the periosteal surface of bone.

The periosteum itself is well supplied by blood vessels; the outer shell of the cortex is normally supplied by capillaries arising from the periosteum, but in senescent and vascularly insufficient specimens the periosteal arteries supply more extensively and deeply into the cortex (Brookes and Revell, 1997). There are extensive anastamoses between the medullary and periosteal circulations, which give the anatomical basis for a flexible blood flow response. It has been suggested that the direction of cortical blood flow depends on the patho-physiological requirement, and the periosteal circulation is acutely capable of responding to injury to the nutrient supply (Reichert, McCarthy and Hughes, 1995).

In Figure 13.1, the arrangement of the vascular system and the diaphyseal cortex is shown. In general, blood flow is centrifugal. Intraosseous vascular pressures are high. It has also been shown that extravascular tissue pressures are high within bone (Wilkes and Visscher, 1975), with a gradient from endosteal to periosteal surface. These high intraossseous pressures are determined by vascular parameters and the hydraulic conductivity of bone. This arrangement of blood flow and pressure appears to be a uniform and general feature of bone and suggests that local control of vascular resistance is an important aspect of the overall functional design of bones.

13.2.2 Microvascular structure in bone

In cortical bone, capillaries are found within the Haversian canal and are, therefore, orientated parallel to the long axis of long bones. Capillary structure can be classified as being continous, fenestrated or discontinuous. Descriptions of capillary structure in dog cortical bone have been made from electron microscopy (Cooper, Milgram and Robinson, 1966). These studies show Haversian canals typically 50–70 μm in diameter; these canals contain one or, occasionally, two capillaries. The capillaries are continuous in structure, that is they have tight junctions.

13.2.3 Perivascular innervation of bone

Bone and periosteum are innervated by both sympathetic and sensory nerves, though innervation is much more dense in the periosteum. As well as noradrenergic sympathetic fibres, peptidergic nerves containing substance P, calcitonin gene-related peptide, vasoactive intestinal peptide and neuropeptide Y have also been described (Bjurholm *et al.*, 1988). Innervation is more dense near the epiphyseal plate, bone marrow and the periosteum. Using protein gene product 9.5, a general neural marker, it has been shown that most nerve fibres in bone marrow, periosteum and cortex are closely associated with blood vessels (Hukkanen *et al.*, 1993).

13.2.4 Adrenergic control

The effects of neurohumeral agents on bone blood flow have been studied, and it has been shown that noradrenaline affects both flow and vascular resistance. However, the most precise measurements of vascular reactivity of bone have been performed in experimental preparations that perfuse the nutrient supply of a long bone, and in which perfusion pressure is continuously monitored to investigate changes in vascular resistance (Driessens and Vanhoutte, 1979). This technique allows precise physiological assessments of changes in the vascular reactivity of bone as a whole but does not provide an insight into the anatomical distribution of relative responses, e.g. major vesssels or arterioles, cortical bone, trabecular bone

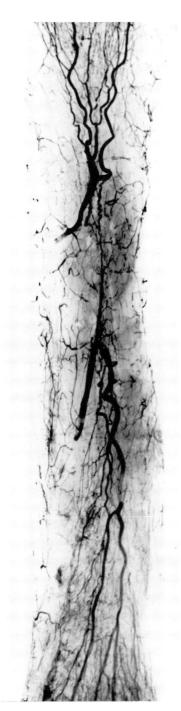

Figure 13.1. Vascular arrangement of the femoral diaphysis of a child, aged eight years. (From H. V. Crock, with permission.)

or marrow. Studies of perivascular innervation of vessels in bone show a very selective distribution. Using the bone perfusion technique, the response of bone to a wide range of vasoactive substances has been investigated by several groups. It has been shown that, in general, the vasculature in bone responds to most vasoconstrictor and vasodilator substances; however, it has been proposed that bone is relatively hypersensitive to vasoconstrictors, when compared with responses in other tissues, and relatively hyposensitive to vasodilators (Brinker *et al.*, 1990).

Recently, experiments have been performed on isolated arteries dissected from both animal bone and human bone. These studies indicate that α_1-receptors are responsible for the constrictive adrenergic response in bone (Lundgaard *et al.*, 1996).

13.2.5 Endothelial-dependent control

The existence of NO-dependent vasodilatation has been documented in bone (Brinker *et al.*, 1990; Davis and Wood, 1992). Brinker and co-workers demonstrated vasodilatation in response to acetylcholine and nitroglycerine (an exogenous source of NO) without demonstrating that acetylcholine acted by the NO pathway. It has also been demonstrated that acetylcholine will diminish the vasoconstrictive effects of noradrenaline, and that this effect is abolished in the presence of an inhibitor of NO production (Davis and Wood, 1992).

Vasodilatation to NO has been demonstrated in bone preparations in experiments from this laboratory (McCarthy *et al.*, 1997) using *ex vivo* isolated perfused tibia preparations. The experimental setup is illustrated in Figure 13.2. The bone is

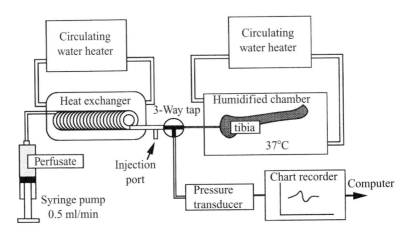

Figure 13.2. Apparatus used for the *ex vivo* perfusion of the rabbit tibia. The tibia is maintained at 37 °C and perfused with Krebs-Ringer buffer (also warmed to 37 °C). Pressure is monitored continuously, and there is an injection port to allow access for the administration of boluses of acetylcholine. Depending on the stage of the experiment, the perfusate may contain noradrenaline to raise the vascular tone or 10^{-4} M L-NAME to inhibit NO synthesis.

perfused at a constant flow rate, and perfusion pressure is monitored continuously. Any changes in perfusion pressure indicate a change in the vascular resistance of the bone. As an isolated preparation such as this is maximally vasodilated, it is necessary to raise the vascular resistance by the addition of a vasoconstrictor to the perfusate, in this case noradrenaline, until the perfusion pressure approaches physiological values. The effect of bolus injections of acetylcholine is shown in Figure 13.3. There is a dose-dependent vasodilatation that is abolished in the presence of L-NAME. This demonstrates that acetylcholine is affecting vasodilatation via an NO-mediated pathway.

13.3 The role of the microcirculation in bone physiology

It has often been noted that angiogenesis preceded osteogenesis in many practical situations, and this empirical observation has led to the suggestion that the blood vessels play an active role in the process of osteogenesis rather than just a passive role of providing substrates for the process of osteogenesis (Trueta, 1963). Recent laboratory studies have given further direct suppport to this hypothesis and also suggested a role for the endothelium and NO in normal skeletal homeostasis.

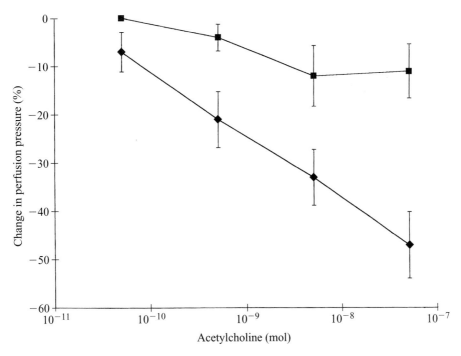

Figure 13.3. The effect of bolus injections of acetylcholine on perfusion pressure in the isolated tibia. Perfusion pressure has been raised to around 100 mmHg by the addition of noradrenaline to the perfusatae. Vasodilatation is significantly diminished when 10^{-4} M L-NAME is added to the perfusate: Krebs media alone (◆); with L-NAME (■).

Villanueva and Nimni (1990) implanted rat fetal calvarial cells and endothelial cells isolated from rat liver or bovine aorta into diffusion chambers placed subcutaneously in rats. The amount of mineralization and alkaline phosphatase activity was very significantly higher in chambers containing both calvarial and endothelial cells, compared with chambers containing either calvarial or endothelial cells. Endothelial cells alone seemed to enhance angiogenesis around the diffusion chambers (Villanueva and Nimni, 1990). Cell culture experiments have demonstrated that isolated microvessel cells (both endothelium and pericytes) have a mitogenic effect on osteoblast-enriched calvarial cells that is mediated by soluble factors (Jones, Clark and Brighton, 1995). It was also shown that the microvessel cells produced a prolonged reduction in the expression of markers of the osteoblast phenotype.

Recent advances in vascular biology show that the endothelium is not a passive barrier between blood and vascular smooth muscle but rather an active tissue in its own right, releasing vasoconstrictor and vasodilator substances and secreting other immunoregulatory factors. It is also a target for circulating hormones and local regulatory factors. It has been shown that vascular endothelial cells produce potential modulators of bone activity such as FGFs, IL-1 and IL-6, CSFs, prostacyclin, endothelin-1 and NO. Vascular endothelial cells cloned from fetal bovine bone have been shown to respond to PTH, progesterone, oestrogen, IGFs, PDGF, basic FGF and endothelial cell growth factor. It has, therefore, been argued that bone vascular endothelial cells should be considered to be an important part of the bone cell communication network (Collin-Osdoby, 1994).

13.3.1 Venous pressure and bone formation

Several studies have indicated that manipulation of the vascular system serving bone can stimulate bone formation and increase the rate of fracture repair. The first reported observation was by Ambroise Pare, and there have been regular reports in the literature since then.

It has been shown by Kelly and co-workers that the application of a venous tourniquet proximal to the knee, with a skin pressure of 30 mmHg, can stimulate periosteal new bone formation in the tibia in puppies in seven days (Kelly and Bronk, 1990) and can increase the rate of fracture repair (Kruse and Kelly, 1974). It was also shown that the venous tourniquet increased intramedullary pressure. Direct increase of intramedullary pressure by infusion through a paediatric cannula has been shown to increase the rate of periosteal bone formation in immature goats (Welch et al., 1993).

Interestingly, recent data on bone mass changes during space flight are now also providing data to demonstrate an association between changes in bone mass and pressure changes. Normally, while standing on the surface of the earth, there is a gradient of pressures within the capillaries, the lowest pressures being in the head, and the highest in the feet. When weightless (or when lying down), this gradient disappears, and capillary pressures are uniform throughout the body. Therefore, capillary pressures in the head increase, pressures in the feet decrease and pressures at the level of the heart remain unchanged. Measurement of bone density after prolonged exposure to microgravity show that bone is lost mainly from the lower limbs, there is little change in bone mass in the trunk, but bones above the level of the heart increase in mass. Some data illustrating this from a recent 6-month space mission are shown in Figure 13.4. It can be seen that there is an association between changes in capillary pressure and bone density; bone density appears to increase in those bones where capillary pressure is reported to increase, and it decreases in those bones where capillary pressure is reported to decrease. These observations are also supported by ground-based studies that simulate weightlessness.

The mechanisms by which this occurs are not fully understood as yet. It has been shown that circulatory pressure gradients can give rise to streaming potentials (Otter, Palmieri and Cochran, 1990). It is possible that bone responds to mechanical load by some consequence of strain, such as shear forces produced by fluid movement, or by potentials generated by fluid movement, and it is interesting to speculate that the response to pressure changes may be acting via the same mechanism as mechanical loads. However, potentials generated by circulatory pressures are much less than those generated by mechanical loads. Both mechanical loads and shear forces result in NO release (Klein-Nuland *et al.*, 1995; Pitsillides *et al.*, 1995), and it is possible that cardiovascular pressure gradients could also stimulate bone formation via an NO-mediated pathway, or that local control of intraosseous pressure by NO could modulate bone mass.

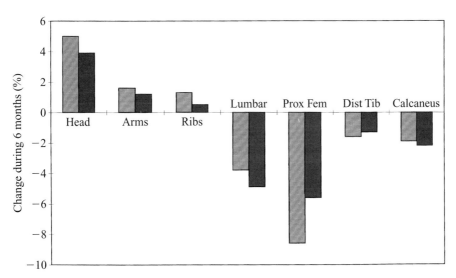

Figure 13.4. Regional changes in bone mineral density measured by dual energy X-ray absorptiometry before (light hatching) and after (dark hatching) a six month period of weightlessness. Prox Fem, proximal femur; Dist Tib, distal tibia.

13.4 Pathophysiology of microcirculation in bone

13.4.1 Ischaemia/reperfusion injury

It is now also becoming accepted that endothelial cells also have an important role in the response of tissue to ischaemia/reperfusion injury (Grace, 1994). Recently, it has been demonstrated not only that normal endothelial cells can have an effect on bone but also that 4.5 h of ischaemia to a hind limb of a rat can produce a periosteal proliferative response 72 h after the ischaemic insult in the tibia of that limb (Svindland *et al.*, 1995). Studies by Wood and co-workers have investigated the response of bone vasculature to periods of ischaemia and found differing responses for different receptor types (Davis and Wood, 1992).

Using an isolated perfused rabbit tibia model, the effect of ischaemia for times of up to 24 h followed by reperfusion with oxygenated Krebs buffer on endothelial-dependent vasodilatation has been investiaged. Acetylcholine produced vasodilatation of the bone vascular bed after the basal tone has been raised by noradrenaline perfusion (Figure 13.3). Vasodilatation was maintained for up to 6 h of warm ischaemia but was abolished after 12 h (Figure 13.5). L-NAME significantly attenuated the vasodilator response to acetylcholine in the early ischaemic stages (less than 6 h). It seems, therefore, that the vasodilatation produced by acetylcholine in this model involved NO synthesis and that this locally mediated regulatory mechanism is irreversibly damaged by ischaemic periods of greater than 12 h.

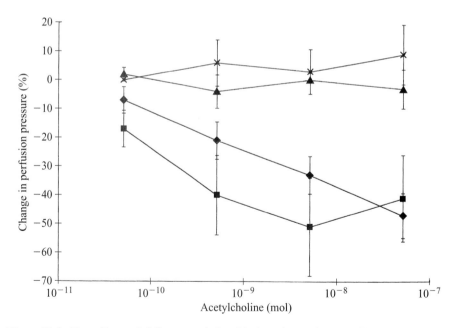

Figure 13.5. The effects of different periods of ischaemia on the vasodilator properties of acetylcholine in an isolated perfused tibia preparation. A vasodilator response is maintained for at least 6 h, but it is abolished after 12 h. Response measured at 0(◆), 6(■), 12(▲) and 24 h(X) of ischaemia.

Histological sections of the nutrient arteries of the tibial preparations showed damage to the endothelium in specimens subjected to ischaemia for longer than 12 h. It is possible that the 'no-reflow' phenomenon observed in these specimens was caused in part by endothelial injury, particularly as the response to noradrenaline was maintained in all the specimens. Whether this injury was caused by ischaemia alone or by ischaemia and reperfusion is not clear. More recent studies suggest that endothelial dysfunction can be inhibited by perfusing the bones with a combination of allopurinol and oxypurinol. However, NO has a possible dual role in ischaemia/reperfusion injury, as NO synthesis may lead to the production of peroxynitrite, a very reactive oxidant that may lead to cell death.

Evaluation of bone allograft preservation techniques using perfusion of cold University of Wisconsin solution at low flow rate has been performed (Moran, Adams and Wood, 1993). Using acetylcholine-dependent vasodilatation as an assay of endothelial viability, it was shown that the integrity of this response can be maintained after five days of cold perfusion with the solution. However, in a subsequent study, vascularized dog tibial allografts preserved in this way for 20 h were transplanted into recipient animals; the response to acetylcholine was a reduction in blood flow, as determined by microsphere injection (Moran *et al.*, 1995). This paradoxical response was inhibited by L-NMMA. It was suggested that the acetylcholine-mediated vasoconstriction seen in these preparations resulted from endothelial dysfunction secondary to reperfusion injury.

13.4.2 Oestrogen receptors in bone

Oestrogen is a potent inhibitor of bone resorption. Loss of ovarian function, such as at the menopause, results in dramatic bone loss. The bone density of a 70-year-old woman can be 30% less than that of a young adult. Post-menopausal bone loss is a significant cause of morbidity in ageing woman, as fracture risk increases exponentially with decreasing bone mineral density.

The mechanism by which oestrogen mediates bone resorption is not entirely clear. Oestrogen receptors have been identified in cells with the osteoblast phenotype, and some recent studies have reported receptors on osteoclasts. It is possible that oestrogen loss results in an IL-6 mediated stimulation of osteoclastogenesis.

It has also been suggested that oestrogen-induced skeletal protection is mediated by the release of NO from bone vascular endothelium as well as bone cells. Oestrogen receptors have been reported on bovine bone endothelial cells (Brandi *et al.*, 1993), and oestrogen stimulated endothelial cell proliferation *in vitro* and also inhibited PTH responsiveness. It was proposed that these obseravations suggested that post-menopausal osteoporosis may be, at least in part, caused by lack of an oestrogen effect directly on bone endothelium. This effect of oestrogen may be mediated by NO, as NO donors abolish overiectomy-induced bone loss (Wimalawansa *et al.*, 1996). Oestradiol therapy in guinea pigs has been shown to increase calcium-dependent NOS activity in several tissues in both males and females. However, ovariectomy has been shown to increase blood flow in rats (Kapitola, Kubickova and Andrle, 1995).

13.4.3 Control of bone blood flow in fracture repair

Bone blood flow increases dramatically in the early stages of fracture healing, both in experimental studies (Paradis and Kelly, 1975) and in clinical investigations (Ashcroft *et al.*, 1992). Blood flow peaks at about 2 weeks after fracture, reaching ten times the flow in normal bone. By 4 weeks, flow has decreased significantly but remains higher than normal for at least 12 weeks.

Fixation techniques can have a considerable effect on the vascular response to fractures. Removal of the periosteum for 2 cm either side of the fracture gap and placing a silicone rubber sheath over the periosteal surface significantly reduced blood flow to the fracture site and effectively produced a fracture non-union (Wallace *et al.*, 1991). This demonstrated the importance of the periosteum in both the vascular response and the overall fracture repair process. More recently, it has been shown that intramedullary reaming alone can stimulate a sixfold increase in periosteal blood flow (Reichert *et al.*, 1995). Both these studies emphasize the importance of maintaining a viable periosteum during fracture fixation. Cortical osteopenia beneath a compression plate may be a result of necrosis, rather than a response to mechanical stress protection (Perren *et al.*, 1988). Micromotion at the fracture site has also been shown to produce a greater vascular response at the fracture site.

Hukkanen and co-workers have demonstrated rapid proliferation of calcitonin gene-related peptide-containing nerves during healing of rat tibial fracture (Hukkanen *et al.*, 1993). These results are consistent with the neural involvement in bone growth and remodelling, and it has, therefore, been postulated that such sensory innervation may have an important role in fracture vascular control, angiogenesis and osteogenesis.

All these studies show the importance of the vascular response in fractures; recently, some experiments have investigated the role of NO in linking the vascular and osteogenic responses. Corbett and co-workers have shown the presence of both eNOS and iNOS at the fracture site of an experimental model (Corbett *et al.*, 1996). This is, potentially, of major importance, as NO has been shown not only to be a potent vasodilator and potential angiogenic stimulus but also to be an important secondary messenger in bone cell metabolism. The demonstration of eNOS in blood vessels about the fracture site in the early stages of repair suggests that these vessels are active in the production of NO, thereby causing vasodilatation and increasing the surface area available for exchange. In addition, the NO generated may then also influence the callus formation and ensuing repair process.

13.5 Conclusions

Although it is commonly perceived that the circulation in bone is relatively unreactive, detailed measurements show considerable control of vascular tone, and there is now good evidence to support an important role for NO in local control of vascular tone. Recent experimental and clinical studies indicate an important role for the microcirculation in bone physiology, either through local control of intraosseous pressures or by paracrine action of bone endothelial cells; both may be mediated by NO.

References

Ashcroft, G. P., Evans, N. T. S., Roeda, D. *et al.* (1992) Measurement of blood flow in tibial fracture patients using positron emission tomography *J. Bone Joint Surg.* **74B**, 673–677.

Bjurholm, A., Kreicbergs, A., Brodin, E. and Schultzberg, M. (1988) Substance P- and CGRP-immunoreactive nerves in bone. *Peptides* **9**, 165–171.

Brandi, M. L., Crescioli, C., Tanini, A., Frediani, U., Agnusdei, D. and Gennari, C. (1993) Bone endothelial cells as estrogen targets. *Calcif. Tiss. Int.* **53**, 312–317.

Brinker, M. R., Lippton, H. L., Cook, S. D. and Hyman, A. L. (1990) Pharmacological regulation of the circulation of bone *J. Bone Joint Surg.* **72A**, 964–975.

Brookes, M. and Revell, W. J. (1997) *The Blood Supply of Bone.* Springer, London.

Collin-Osdoby, P. (1994) Role of vascular endothelial cells in bone biology. *J. Cell Biochem.* **55**, 304–309.

Cooper, R. R., Milgram, J. W. and Robinson, R. A. (1966) Morphology of the osteon. An electron microscope study. *J. Bone Joint Surg.* **48A**, 1239–1271.

Corbett, S. A., Hukkanen, M., McCarthy, I. D., Polak, J. M. and Hughes, S. P. F. (1996) Expression of nitric oxide synthase isoforms in rat tibial fracture callus. *J. Bone Joint Surg.* **79B** (Suppl. IV), 468.

Crock, H. V. (1996) *An Atlas of Vascular Anatomy of the Skeleton and Spinal Cord.* Martin Dunitz, London.

Davis, T. R. C. and Wood, M. B. (1992) Endothelial control of long bone vascular resistance. *J. Orthop. Res.* **10**, 344–349.

Driessens, M. and Vanhoutte, P. M. (1979) Vascular reactivity of the isolated tibia of the dog. *Am. J. Physiol.* **236**, H904–H908.

Grace, P. A. (1994) Ischaemia–reperfusion injury. *Br. J. Surg.* **81**, 637–647.

Hukkanen, M., Konttinen, Y. T., Santavirta, S. *et al.* (1993) Rapid proliferation of calcitonic gene-related peptide-immunoreactive nerves during healing of rat tibial fracture suggests neural involvement in bone growth and remodelling. *Neuroscience* **54**, 969–979.

Jones, A. R., Clark, C. C. and Brighton, C. T. (1995) Microvessel endothelial cells and pericytes increase proliferation and repress osteoblast phenotypic markers in rat calvarial bone cell cultures. *J. Orthop. Res.* **13**, 553–561.

Kapitola, J., Kubickova, J. and Andrle, J. (1995) Blood flow and mineral content of the tibia of female and male rats: changes following castration and/or administration of estradiol or testosterone. *Bone* **16**, 69–72.

Kelly, P. J. and Bronk, J. T. (1990) Venous pressure and bone formation. *Microvasc. Res.* **39**, 364–375.

Klein-Nuland, J., Semeins, C. M., Ajubi, N. E., Nijweide, P. J. and Burger, E. H. (1995) Pulsating fluid flow increases nitric oxide (NO) synthesis by osteocytes but not periosteal fibroblasts – correlation with prostaglandin up-regulation. *Biochim. Biophys. Res. Commun.* **217**, 640–648.

Kruse, R. L. and Kelly, P. J. (1974) Acceleration of fracture healing distal to a venous tourniquet. *J. Bone Joint Surg.* **56A**, 730–739.

Lundgaard, A., Aslkjaer, C. and Hansen, E. B. (1996) First report on vascular reactivity in human bone tissue. In *7th Int. Symp. Bone Necrosis,* Fukuoka.

McCarthy, I. D., Andhoga, M., Batten, J. J. and Mathie, R. T. (1997) Endothelium-dependent vasodilatation produced by the L-arginine/nitrite oxide pathway in normal and ischaemic bone. *Acta Orthop. Scand.,* **68**, 361–368.

Moran, C. G., Adams, M. L. and Wood, M. B. (1993) Preservation of bone graft vascularity with the University of Wisconsin cold storage solution. *J. Orthop. Res.* **11**, 840–848.

Moran, C. G., McGrory, B. J., Bronk, J. T. and Wood, M. B. (1995) Reperfusion injury in vascularized bone allografts. *J. Orthop. Res.* **13**, 368–374.

Otter, M. W., Palmieri, V. R. and Cochran, G. V. B. (1990) Transcortical streaming potentials are generated by circulatory pressure gradients in living canine tibia. *J. Orthop Res.* **8**, 119–126.

Paradis, G. R. and Kelly, P. J. (1975) Blood flow and mineral deposition in canine tibial fractures. *J. Bone Joint Surg.* **57A**, 220–226.

Perren, S. M., Cordey, J., Rahn, B. A., Gautier, E. and Schneider, E. (1988) Early temporary porosis of bone induced by internal fixation of implants. *Clin. Orthop. Rel. Res.* **232**, 139–151.

Pitsillides, A. A., Rawlinson, S. C. F., Suswillo, F. L., Bourine, S., Zaman, G. and Lanyon, L. E. (1995) Mechanical strain-induced NO production by bone cells: a possible role in adaptive (re)modeling. *FASEB J.* **9**, 1614–1622.

Reichert, I. L. H., McCarthy, I. D. and Hughes, S. P. F. (1995) The acute vascular response to intramedullary reaming. *J. Bone Joint Surg.* **77B**, 490–493.

Svindland, A. D., Nordfletten, S., Reikeraf, F. and Skjeldal, F. (1995) Periosteal response to transient ischaemia: histological studies on rat tibia. *Acta Orthop. Scand.* **66**, 468–472.

Trueta, J. (1963) The role of the vessels in osteogenesis. *J. Bone Joint Surg.* **45B**, 402–418.

Villanueva, J. E. and Nimni, M. E. (1990) Promotion of calvarial cell osteogenesis by endothelial cells. *J. Bone Min. Res.* **5**, 733–739.

Wallace, A. L., Draper, E. R. C., Strachan, R. K., McCarthy, I. D. and Hughes, S. P. F. (1991) The effect of devascularisation upon early bone healing in dynamic external fixation. *J. Bone Joint Surg.* **73B**, 819–825.

Welch, R. D., Johnston, C. E., Waldron, M. J. and Potet, B. (1993) Bone changes associated with intraosseous hypertension in the caprine tibia. *J. Bone Joint Surg.* **75A**, 53–60.

Wilkes, C. H. and Visscher, M. B. (1975) Some physiological aspects of bone marrow pressure. *J. Bone Joint Surg.* **57A**, 49–56.

Wimalawansa, S. J., De Marco, G., Gangula, P. and Yallampalli, C. (1996) Nitric acid donor alleviates ovariectomy-induced bone loss. *Bone* **18**, 301–304.

14

Fluid shear stress

TODD N. MCALLISTER and JOHN A. FRANGOS

14.1 Introduction

Maintenance of the skeletal system is controlled by a complex system of mechanical and biochemical signals that metabolically optimize mineral homeostasis and mechanical integrity. It is well known that physiological bone maintenance and remodelling is mediated by the local mechanical environment (Frost, 1964; Wolff, 1986). This is best illustrated by examples of disuse osteoporosis. Reduced mechanical loading associated with microgravity, head down tilt (cephalad fluid shift) or extended bedrest results in resorptive activity and substantial loss of bone mass. Within hours of exposure to microgravity, resorptive activity results in marked increases in blood calcium levels and in other markers of resorptive activity (Tilton, Degioanni, and Schneider, 1980; Hargens et al., 1983; Arnaud et al., 1988; Roer and Dillaman, 1990). Similarly, orthopaedic implant failure is frequently associated with localized resorption in areas of stress shielding (Harris, 1992; Huiskes, Weinans and van Rietbergen, 1992).

Conversely, athletes demonstrate increased bone mass associated with increased skeletal loading (Suominen, 1993). There are several studies which show that critically sized open fractures can be induced to close using elastic or hydraulic fixators that allow a small amount of relative motion at the fracture site (Goodship et al., 1993; Claes et al., 1995). Interestingly, the skeletal system in nearly all species experiences maximal physiological strains of the order of 3000 $\mu\varepsilon$ (microstrain), suggesting a common mechanism that mediates the response to loading (Rubin, McLeod and Bain, 1990).

Despite the prevalence of examples of mechanically mediated bone maintenance, little is known about the pathways responsible for converting mechanical input into mitogenic or resorptive signals. The role of fluid flow in this mechanochemical signal transduction was recognized in the medical literature in the 1500s, when venous stasis was a noted treatment for fracture repair and orthopaedic pathogenesis (Malgaigne, 1840). Likewise, changes in intraosseous pressure associated with arteriovenous aneurysms in the femoral or inguinal region resulted in significant leg lengthening compared with normal contralateral limbs. Moreover, venous stasis was successfully utilized in the normal limbs to match the increased length. These empirical results were studied in more detail in 1930 using a canine model (Pearse and Morton, 1930). Defects were introduced into both fibulae of adult dogs, then the popliteal vein in one limb was ligated to induce venous stasis. The dogs were left to ambulate normally, and in all but one case the ligated limb repaired more rapidly and with a higher degree of stability. Although these circulatory anomalies were clearly associated with osteogenesis, they were originally attributed to increased carbon dioxide and decreased pH associated with stasis. More recently, investigators have associated this osteogenic response with increases in intraosseous pressure. Using a canine model, localized remodelling was associated with ligation or tourniquet-induced venous occlusion. The increases in transmural pressure associated with extended venous stasis were demonstrated to stimulate significant periosteal bone deposition (Kelly, 1968; Kelly and Bronk, 1990). Using a rabbit model, venous occlusion was shown to increase intraosseous pressure and augment load-induced transients in the medullary cavity (Beverly, Pflug and Mathie, 1987). A relationship was noted between intraosseous pressure, loading and periosteal drainage, suggesting that bone behaved like a compressible, perfused sponge. Likewise, studies with cephalad fluid shifts from extended head-down tilt demonstrated reduced cortical thickness in the femur, as would be expected with disuse osteoporosis. Surprisingly, the increased medullary pressure associated with the fluid shift increased bone mass in the mandible and skull (Roer and Dillaman, 1990). These studies are notable in that the bone remodelling was triggered by factors independent of mechanical strain. In each of these examples, fluid flow was altered by changes in the intraosseous venous pressure in the absence of changes in mechanical loading. This suggests that fluid flow is an important parameter in bone maintenance and remodelling. Despite these early observations, the role of fluid flow in the physiology of bone turnover has been largely ignored. Recent studies, however, demonstrate a significant role for fluid flow in mechanotransduction and hormonal control of bone remodelling.

14.2 Fluid flow in bone

Bone is a porous medium with up to 22% total void volume and is characterized by three levels of porosity (Black and Mattson, 1982; McCarthy and Yang, 1992; Weinbaum, Cowin and Zeng, 1994). The canaliculi make up the intermediate level of porosity and account for approximately 10–15% of the total porosity in bone (Black and Mattson, 1982; McCarthy and Yang, 1992). This network has been shown to facilitate substantial and rapid transcortical interstitial fluid (ISF) flow (Anderson, 1960; Frost, 1964; Seliger, 1969; Johnson et al., 1982; Kelly, 1983; Dillaman, 1984; Montgomery et al., 1988; Kelly, Montgomery and Bronk, 1990; Kufahl and Saha, 1990; Dillaman, Roer and Gay, 1991; Weinbaum et al., 1994; Keanini, Roer and Dillaman, 1995). Osteocytes extend processes through the canaliculi and are connected via gap junctions, suggesting a communicating network throughout the cortex.

Interstitial fluid flow originates from leaky venous sinusoids in the intramedullary cavity and is driven radially outward through cortical bone by a transmural pressure gradient between the endosteal vasculature and the lymphatic drainage at the periosteal surface (Seliger, 1969; Kelly, 1983; Dillaman, 1984; Dillaman *et al.*, 1991). In the absence of mechanical loading, this flow is relatively steady with only minor oscillations associated with pulse (Otter, Palmieri and Cochran, 1990). Mechanical strain from locomotion or posture maintenance generates pulsatile flow associated with both the loading and concomitant relaxation. Like stepping on a sponge, localized pressure gradients arise from bending or compressive loads, driving fluid from areas of compression to other areas where tension increases (Otter *et al.*, 1996). Torsional loads, however, do not induce significant flow. Approximately 80% of physiological loading is carried in bending (Rubin *et al.*, 1990).

Interstitial fluid flow has been characterized indirectly through a series of *in vivo* studies. Using markers such as thorium dioxide, ferritin and horse radish peroxidase, investigators have demonstrated a rapid fluid efflux from the endosteum to the periosteal surface (Seliger, 1969; Dillaman, 1984; Montgomery *et al.*, 1988; Dillaman *et al.*, 1991; Keanini *et al.*, 1995). Likewise, Otter has demonstrated the presence of a streaming potential in bone that is derived from electrolytic interstitial fluid flowing across a charged surface (Otter *et al.*, 1990, 1996). It is important to note, however, that these studies offer only indirect evidence of the characteristics and effects of interstitial flow. Although theoretical studies suggest that this flow generates fluid shear stresses of the same order of magnitude as the vascular system ($8-30$ dyne/cm^2), no direct measurement has yet been made in bone (Weinbaum *et al.*, 1994).

14.3 Mechanisms of flow-mediated remodelling

Based on these investigations and observations, it is clear that fluid flow plays an important role in bone remodelling. In an effort to elucidate the mechanisms of fluid flow-induced remodelling and to aid in defining clinically relevant treatment strategies, several *in vitro* studies have been conducted. Most of these investigations focus on either flow-induced streaming potentials or flow-induced shear stresses.

In 1990, we hypothesized that fluid flow-induced shear stresses mediate bone remodelling (Reich, Gay and Frangos, 1990). Using well-defined fluid flow profiles, investigators have demonstrated flow to be a potent stimulus of autocrine/pararine factors that affect the migration, proliferation and activation of osteoclasts, osteoblasts and osteocytes. Specifically, flow has been shown to stimulate inositol 1,4,5-triphosphate (IP$_3$), cAMP, prostaglandins E$_2$, I$_2$ and G/H, TGFβ and calcium in osteoblasts, and prostoglandin E$_2$ production in osteocytes (Reich *et al.*, 1990, 1997; Reich and Frangos, 1991; Reich, 1993; Klein-Nulend *et al.*, 1995, 1996a). More recently, investigators have demonstrated flow-induced NO production in osteoblasts and osteocytes (Johnson, McAllister and Frangos, 1996; Klein-Nulend *et al.*, 1996b).

NO has been shown to mediate bone remodelling by inhibiting osteoclastic resorption (MacIntyre *et al.*, 1991; Kasten *et al.*, 1994; Collin-Osdoby, Nickols and Osdoby, 1995). Moreover, NO has been shown to have a dose-dependent bi-phasic effect on osteoblast activity, suggesting an autoregulated control system (Riancho *et al.*, 1995a, b). It is likely, however, that osteoclast inhibition dominates the NO-mediated effects. Osteoclasts migrate and resorb bone at three to five times the rate of osteoblast deposition. This suggests that osteoclast inhibition would have a more rapid and pronounced effect than osteoblast stimulation.

Using a well-defined shear stress of 6 dyne/cm^2 in a parallel plate flow chamber and constant head recirculating flow loop, we have demonstrated rapid and continuous release of NO in primary rat calvarial osteoblasts (Johnson *et al.*, 1996). This synthesis was inhibited with L-arginine analogues, but dexamethasone, which inhibits iNOS induction, had no significant effect. This suggests that the NO was derived from a constitutively present NOS isoform. While several investigators have used cytokines to induce NO release (Lowik *et al.*, 1994; Hukkanen *et al.*, 1995; Riancho *et al.*, 1995b) and others have shown induction of iNOS mRNA (Ralston *et al.*, 1994; Riancho *et al.*, 1995a), this was the first report of a constitutively present and functional NOS isoform in bone. While the cytokine studies indicate that osteoblasts are capable of producing iNOS, it is not clear which isoform is constitutively present. PCR techniques have demonstrated nNOS mRNA in osteo-blasts, but, to date, no study has definitively identified the functional isoform in osteoblasts or osteocytes (Pitsillides *et al.*, 1995; Riancho *et al.*, 1995a).

14.4 Streaming potentials

The observations discussed above suggest a role for fluid flow in mechanochemical signal transduction but do not distinguish between streaming potential- or shear stress-mediated effects. Flow-induced streaming potentials are generated by an electrolytic fluid moving over a charged surface, and this electric potential has been proposed to mediate localized bone remodelling. Interstitial fluid flow in a bone loaded in bending generates flow from the concave surface toward the convex surface and, therefore, develops a positive charge on the convex surface. Osteoblasts have been shown to migrate preferentially to negatively charged surfaces and osteoclasts have been shown to migrate preferentially to positively charged surfaces (Ferrier, Ross and Kanehisa, 1986). This selective electrokinetic migration serves as the basis for streaming potential-mediated remodelling theories.

Streaming potentials are a function of the electrochemical properties of the fluid and of the surface over which it flows as well as of the fluid velocity. Shear stress, unlike streaming potentials, varies proportionally with viscosity. In an effort to discriminate fluid flow-induced shear stress effects from effects owing to streaming potentials, flow-induced cAMP responses were monitored using different fluid viscosities. The cAMP response was shown to be viscosity dependent, suggesting that fluid shear stresses and not streaming potentials mediated the cAMP response (Reich *et al.*, 1990). Likewise, the mechanisms of flow-mediated stimulation of intracellular calcium in osteoblasts have been investigated (Williams *et al.*, 1994;

Hung *et al.*, 1995, 1996). By applying an external countercurrent to negate or enhance the effects of the flow-induced streaming potential, Hung and co-workers demonstrated that the mean peak calcium response was unaltered by either cancelling or doubling the electrokinetic forces (Hung *et al.*, 1996). This suggests that fluid shear stress and not the concomitant electric potential mediates intracellular calcium increases with flow in osteoblasts.

There are numerous *in vivo* and *in vitro* reports that suggest that electric fields may affect bone cells and thereby stimulate fracture repair (Becker and Eriksson, 1968; Lavine and Grodzinsky, 1987; McLeod, Lee and Ehrlich, 1987). These reports are difficult to interpret clearly, and to date, no electrical device has been shown unequivocally to affect bone mitogenesis. Taken together, these observations suggest a minimal role for flow-induced streaming potentials.

14.5 Mechanochemical signal transduction

Recent evidence provides compelling evidence for the role of fluid flow-induced shear stresses in mechanotransduction. Fluid shear stress activated G-proteins that were reconstituted into liposomes in the absence of all other cellular components or receptors (Gudi, Nolan and Frangos, 1998). G-proteins have also been implicated in bone remodelling via PGE_2 release. Flow-induced PGE_2 production is pertussis toxin sensitive, suggesting a role for G-proteins in flow-mediated production of autocrine/paracrine factors (Reich *et al.*, 1997). Likewise, unpublished data from our laboratory demonstrates GTPγS treatment (a general G-protein activator) stimulates dose-dependent NO release in rat calvarial osteoblasts as well as in rat and mouse osteosarcoma cell lines. Taken together, these studies demonstrate that fluid shear stresses mediate flow-induced stimulation of bone remodelling in a G-protein-dependent pathway.

14.6 Hormonal control

Transcortical fluid flow is a function of the pressure differential between the intramedullary cavity and the lymphatics at the periosteal surface and of the overall resistance to flow. The resistance to flow is determined by the characteristics of the cortical porosity and the hydraulic conductivity of the bone-lining membrane at the endosteal surface. Osteoblasts and osteoblast-like cells on the endosteal surface of the intramedullary compartment form a membrane that significantly decreases interstitial fluid transport across the cortex. While the resistance resulting from porosity does not change significantly over short periods of time, the permeability of the endosteal membrane has been shown to vary acutely with hormonal treatment (Hillsley and Frangos, 1996).

PTH is known to stimulate osteoclast recruitment and activity (Uy *et al.*, 1995). PTH has also been shown to affect osteoblast morphology and may, therefore be involved with the regulation of transmural fluid flow across the endosteal lining (Tram *et al.*, 1993; Hillsley and Frangos, 1996). We have shown that PTH decreases the hydraulic conductivity of this membrane, thus decreasing transcortical flow and the subsequent flow-mediated signalling factors.

Calcitonin also affected membrane hydraulic conductivity (Hillsley and Frangos, 1996). At low concentrations (100 nM), calcitonin decreased permeability, while at higher concentrations membrane permeability increased, indicating a bi-phasic dose-dependent response. Taken together, these observations suggest a novel mechanism for fluid flow regulation and an additional role for hormonal control in the complex system of bone maintenance and remodelling.

14.7 Sensitivity to different flow parameters

The studies described above demonstrate that fluid flow and flow-induced shear stresses play a significant role in bone turnover. No distinction has been made, however, in the relative sensitivity to different flow parameters. Physiological fluid flow is dynamic, and, over any given period, cells will be subjected to both steady components and pulsatile components that vary in location, magnitude, frequency and rate of change. There is a wide range of physiological shear-stress amplitudes and shear-stress transients associated with different loading regimens. Locomotion is associated with a high-amplitude, low-frequency strain, while posture mainte-nance is associated with a high-frequency, low-amplitude strain. Both are super-imposed onto the baseline steady flow driven by vascular pressure alone. *In vivo* studies with equine tibia demonstrate low-amplitude, high-frequency (20–30 Hz) strains; the signal is thought to be derived from muscle loading during normal posture maintenance. *In vivo* studies with the turkey ulna model demonstrated an osteogenic response to high-frequency low-amplitude input (McLeod, Bain and Rubin, 1990; Rubin *et al.*, 1990). While these studies appear to indicate a frequency dependence, frequency per se may not mediate remodelling activity.

In the vascular system, endothelial cells demonstrate dramatic sensitivity to temporal gradients in shear stress (Noris *et al.*, 1995). By subjecting cells to a pulsatile flow with either sinusoidal (low rate of change) or square wave (high rate of change) input, investigators discriminated between frequency (Hz) and rate of change of shear (dyne/cm^2 per s). It is likely that bone cells have different sensitivities to these parameters as well. Preliminary data in our laboratory shows that osteoblasts respond to impulses in flow more dramatically than to ramped flow to the same magnitude. Northern blot analysis of c-*fos* expression, an indicator of mitogenic activity, showed a 10-fold increase in GAPDH normalized activity for impulse versus ramp flow (X. P. Bao and J. A. Frangos, unpublished data). To fully investigate the role of pulsatile flow and shear rate sensitivity, it is imperative to develop a well-defined model. To date, no such model has been designed.

Taken together, these studies suggest that shear-stress transients may be an important parameter in flow-induced osteogenesis. Steady flow may mediate localized remodelling by inhibiting resorption through regulatory agents such as NO, while pulsatile flow, or transients in shear, mediate new bone formation and deposition by activating mitogenic indicators such as c-*fos*.

14.8 Mechanical strain versus fluid flow

It is difficult to develop *in vivo* models that distinguish between strain and flow effects, but several studies provide evidence for a role for fluid flow in bone remodelling. Investigators have conducted a variety of experiments on strain-induced remodelling using the turkey ulna model. As described earlier, many of these *in vivo* studies do not distinguish between mechanical strain and strain-induced fluid flow. A recent study, however, provides indirect evidence for the importance of flow in these models. Remodelling activity, as measured by periosteal deposition and pore formation, was monitored in axially and torsionally loaded turkey ulnae and compared with contralateral controls. Axial loading, in addition to the axial strain, induces substantial fluid flow. Torsional loading, conversely, will strain the cells without developing a concomitant pressure gradient to drive transcortical flow. This investigation demonstrated that axial loading increased remodelling while torsional loading did not (Rubin *et al.*, 1996).

Likewise, recent *in vitro* investigations designed to differentiate strain and flow effects demonstrate that flow is the primary remodelling signal in osteoblasts (Owan *et al.*, 1997). Using a four-point bending apparatus submerged in culture media, osteoblasts were mechanically strained. The relative motion of the plate in the liquid media develops fluid forces that are proportional to the velocity of the plate (loading frequency). The mechanical strain in this model is directly proportional to the plate thickness (distance from the neutral axis). Therefore, for any given loading frequency, the fluid forces were varied by changing the overall deflection while the strain was kept constant by changing the plate thickness. Osteopontin expression was used as an indicator of remodelling activity over three ranges of physiological strain and strain rate. Although the fluid forces are not well defined in this system, this study showed that flow and not mechanical strain stimulated osteoblasts.

14.9 Conclusions

Transcortical fluid flow in bone is regulated by mechanical loading, vascular pressure and calcitrophic hormones. Flow has been shown to be a potent stimulus of a variety of autocrine/paracrine agents that selectively modulate activation, migration and proliferation of bone cells. Fluid flow, therefore, plays an important role in the complex system of bone maintenance and remodelling. Moreover, these studies demonstrate the relevance of fluid flow in clinical settings in orthopaedic pathogenesis. Fluid flow may be an important parameter that has largely been ignored in the osseointegration of surgical implants, in fracture repair and in the treatment of diseases that affect the porosity of bone, such as osteoporosis.

References

Anderson, D. W. (1960) Studies of the lymphatic pathways of bone and bone marrow. *J. Bone Joint Surg.* **42A**, 716–717.

Arnaud, S. B., Powell, M. R., Vernikos-Danellis, J. and Buchanan, J. (1988) Bone mineral and body composition after 30 day head down tilt bedrest. *J. Bone Min. Res.* **3**, S119.

Becker, R. O. and Eriksson, C. (1968) Electrical properties of wet collagen. *Nature* **218**, 166–168.

Beverly, M. C., Pflug, J. J. and Mathie, R. T. (1987) Bone is a flexible perfused sponge? *J. Bone Joint Surg.* **69B**, 494.

Black, J. and Mattson, R. U. (1982) Relationship between porosity and mineralization in the Haversian osteon. *Calcif. Tiss. Int.* **34**, 332–336.

Claes, L., Braun, H., Heitemeyer, U. and Hierholzer, G. (1995) The importance of stability for the healing of comminuted fractures (Abstract). *Trans. Comb. Orthop. Res. Soc.* p. 13.

Collin-Osdoby, P., Nickols, G. A. and Osdoby, P. (1995) Bone cell function, regulation, and communication: a role for nitric oxide. *J. Cell Biochem.* **57**, 399–408.

Dillaman, R. M. (1984) Movement of ferritin in the 2-day-old chick femur. *Anatom. Rec.* **209**, 445–453.

Dillaman, R. M., Roer, R. D. and Gay, D. M. (1991) Fluid movement in bone: theoretical and empirical. *J. Biomechan.* **24**(Suppl. 1), 163–177.

Ferrier, J., Ross, S. M. and Kanehisa, J. (1986) Osteoclasts and osteoblasts migrate in opposite directions in response to a constant electric field. *J. Cell Physiol.* **129**, 283–288.

Frost, H. M. (1964) *Laws of Bone Structure*. Charles C. Thomas, Springfields, IL.

Goodship, A. E., Watkins, P. E., Rigby, H. S. and Kenwright, J. (1993) The role of fixator frame stiffness in the control of fracture healing: an experimental study. *J. Biomechan.* **26**, 1027–1035.

Gudi, S. R. P., Nolan, J. P. and Frangos, J. A. (1998) Modulation of GTPase activity of G proteins by fluid shear stress and phospholipid composition. *Proc. Natl. Acad. Sci., USA* **95**, 2515–2519.

Hargens, A. R., Tipton, C. M., Gollnick, P. D., Mubarak, S. J., Tucker, B. J. and Akeson, W. M. (1983) Fluid shifts and muscle function in humans during acute simulated weightlessness. *J. Appl. Physiol.* **54**, 1003–1009.

Harris, W. H. (1992) Will stress shielding limit the longevity of cemented femoral components of total hip replacement? *Clin. Orthop. Rel. Res.* **274**, 120–123.

Hillsley, M. V. and Frangos, J. A. (1996) Osteoblast hydraulic conductivity is regulated by calcitonin and parathyroid hormone. *J. Bone Min. Res.* **11**, 114–124.

Huiskes, R., Weinans, H. and van Rietbergen, B. (1992) The relationship between stress shielding and bone resorption around total hip stems and the effects of flexible materials. *Clin. Orthop. Rel. Res.* **274**, 124–134.

Hukkanen, M., Hughes, F. J., Buttery, L. D. K. *et al.* (1995) Cytokine-stimulated expression of inducible nitric oxide synthase by mouse, rat, and human osteoblast-like cells and its functional role in osteoblast metabolic activity. *Endocrinology* **136**, 5445–5453.

Hung, C. T., Pollack, S. R., Reilly, T. M. and Brighton, C. T. (1995) Real time calcium response of cultured bone cells to fluid flow. *Clin. Orthop.* **313**, 256–259.

Hung, C. T., Allen, F. D., Pollack, S. R. and Brighton, C. T. (1996) What is the role of the convective current density in the real time calcium response of cultured bone cells to fluid flow. *J. Biomech.* **29**, 1403–1409.

Johnson, D. L., McAllister, T. N. and Frangos, J. A. (1996) Fluid flow stimulates rapid and continuous release of nitric oxide in osteoblasts. *Am. J. Physiol.* **271**, E205–E208.

Johnson, M. W., Chakkalakal, D. A., Harper, R. A. and Katz, J. L. (1982) Fluid flow in bone *in vitro*. *J. Biomechan.* **15**, 881–885.

Kasten, T. P., Collin-Osdoby, P., Patel, N. *et al.* (1994) Potentiation of osteoclast bone resorption activity by inhibition of nitric oxide synthase. *Proc. Natl. Acad. Sci., USA* **91**, 3569–3573.

Keanini, R. G., Roer, R. D. and Dillaman, R. M. (1995) A theoretical model of circulatory interstitial fluid flow and species transport within porous cortical bone. *J. Biomechan.* **28**, 901–914.

Kelly, P. J. (1968) Effect of unilateral increased venous pressure on bone remodeling in canine tibia. *J. Lab. Clin. Med.* **72**, 410–418.

Kelly, P. J. (1983) Pathways of transport in bone. In *Handbook of Physiology*, Section 2: *The Cardiovascular System*, Vol. 3, Part 2 *The Peripheral Circulation* (ed. J. T. Shepherd, F. M. Abboud and S. R. Geiger), pp. 371–396. Williams and Wilkins, Bethesda, MD.

Kelly, P. J. and Bronk, J. T. (1990) Venous pressure and bone formation. *Microvasc. Res.* **39**, 364–375.

Kelly, P. J., Montgomery, R. J. and Bronk, J. T. (1990) Reaction of the circulatory system to injury and regeneration. *Clin. Orthop. Rel. Res.* **254**, 275–288.

Klein-Nulend, J., van der Plas, A., Semeins, C. M. *et al.* (1995) Sensitivity of osteocytes to biomechanical stress *in vitro*. *FASEB J.* **9**, 441–445.

Klein-Nulend, J., Semeins, C. M. and Berger, E. H. (1996a) Prostaglandin mediated modulation of transforming growth factor-beta metabolism in primary mouse osteoblastic cells *in vitro*. *J. Cell Physiol.* **168**, 1–7.

Klein-Nulend, J., Semeins, C. M., Ajubi, N. E., Nijweide, P. J. and Berger, E. H. (1996b) Pulsating fluid flow increases nitric oxide synthesis by osteocytes but not periosteal fibroblasts – correlation with prostaglandin up-regulation. *Biochem. Biophys. Res. Commun.* **217**, 640–648.

Kufahl, R. H. and Saha, S. (1990) A theoretical model for stress-generated fluid flow in the canaliculi–lacunae network in bone tissue. *J. Biomechan.* **23**, 171–180.

Lavine, L. S. and Grodzinsky, A. J. (1987) Electrical stimulation of repair of bone. *J. Bone Joint Surg.* **69A**, 626–630.

Lowik, C. W., Nibbering, P. H., van de Ruit, M. and Papapoulos, S. E. (1994) Inducible production of nitric oxide in osteoblast-like cells and in fetal mouse bone explants is associated with suppression of osteoclastic bone resorption. *J. Clin. Invest.* **93**, 1465–1472.

MacIntyre, I., Zaidi, M., Towhidul Alam, A. S. and Datta, H. K. (1991) Osteoclastic inhibition: an action of nitric oxide not mediated by cyclic GMP. *Proc. Natl. Acad. Sci., USA* **88**, 2936–2940.

Malgaigne, J. F. II (1840) Oeuvres completes d'Ambroise Pare. Paris.

McCarthy, I. D. and Yang, L. (1992) A distributed model of exchange processes within the osteon. *J. Biomechan.* **25**, 441–450.

McLeod, K. J., Lee, R. C. and Ehrlich, H. P. (1987) Frequency dependence of electric field modulation of fibroblast protein synthesis. *Science* **236**, 1465–1469.

McLeod, K. J., Bain, S. D. and Rubin, C. T. (1990) Dependence of bone adaptation on the frequency of induced dynamic strain. *Proc. Orthop. Res. Soc.* p. 103.

Montgomery, R. J., Sutker, B. D., Bronk, J. T., Smith, S. R. and Kelly, P. J. (1988) Interstitial fluid flow in cortical bone. *Microvasc. Res.* **35**, 295–307.

Noris, M., Morigi, M., Donadelli, R. *et al.* (1995) Nitric oxide synthesis by cultured endothelial cells is modulated by flow conditions. *Circ. Res.* **76**, 536–543.

Otter, M. W., Palmieri, V. R. and Cochran, G. V. B. (1990) Transcortical streaming potentials are generated by circulatory pressure gradients in living canine tibia. *J. Orthop. Res.* **8**, 119–126.

Otter, M. W., Bronk, J. T., Wu, D. D., Bieber, W. A., Kelly, P. J. and Cochran, G. V. B. (1996) Inflatable brace-related streaming potentials in living canine tibias. *Clin. Orthop. Rel. Res.* **324**, 283–291.

Owan, I., Burr, D. C., Turner, C. H. *et al.* (1997) Osteoblasts do not respond ro physiological strain but are responsive to fluid effects. *Proc. Orthop. Res. Soc.*, Paper 176.

Pearse, H. E. and Morton, J. J. (1930) The stimulation of bone growth by venous stasis. *J. Bone Joint Surg.* **12**, 97–111.

Pitsillides, A. A., Rawlinson, S. C. F., Suswillo, R. F. L., Zaman, G., Nijweide, P. I. and Lanyon, L. E. (1995) Mechanical strain induced nitric production by osteoblasts osteocytes (Abstract). *J. Bone Min. Res.* **10**, S266.

Ralston, S. H., Todd, D., Helfrich, M., Benjamin, N. and Grabowski, P. S. (1994) Human osteoblast-like cells produce nitric oxide and express inducible nitric oxide synthase. *Endocrinology* **135**, 330–336.

Reich, K. M. (1993) Fluid flow induced signal transduction in osteoblasts. Thesis, Pennsylvania State University.

Reich, K. M. and Frangos, J. A. (1991) Effect of flow on prostaglandin E$_2$ and inositol trisphosphate levels in osteoblasts. *Am. J. Physiol.* **261**(Cell Physiol. **30**), C428–C432.

Reich, K. M., Gay, C. V. and Frangos, J. A. (1990) Fluid shear stress as a mediator of osteoblast cyclic adenosine monophosphate production. *J. Cell Physiol.* **143**, 100–104.

Reich, K. M., McAllister, T. N., Gudi, S. and Frangos, J. A. (1997) Activation of G proteins mediates flow-induced prostaglandin E$_2$ production in osteoblasts. *Endocrinology*, **138**, 1014–1018.

Riancho, J. A., Salas, E., Zarrabeitia, M. T. *et al.* (1995a) Expression and functional role of nitric oxide synthase in osteoblast like cells. *J. Bone Min. Res.* **10**, 439–446.

Riancho, J. A., Zarrabeitia, M. T., Fernandez-Luna, J. L. and Gonzalez-Macias, J. (1995b) Mechanisms controlling nitric oxide synthesis in osteoblasts. *Mol. Cell Endocrinol.* **107**, 87–92.

Roer, R. D. and Dillaman, R. M. (1990) Bone growth and calcium balance during simulated weightlessness in the rat. *J. Appl. Physiol.* **68**, 13–20.

Rubin, C. T., McLeod, K. J. and Bain, S. D. (1990) Functional strains and cortical bone adaptation; epigenetic assurance of skeletal integrity. *J. Biomechan.* **23**, 43–54.

Rubin, C., Gross, T., Qin, Y. X., Fritton, S., Guilak, F. and McLeod, K. (1996) Differentiation of the bone-tissue remodeling response to axial and torsional loading in the turkey ulna. *J. Bone Joint Surg.* **78A**, 1523–1533.

Seliger, W. G. (1969) Tissue fluid movement in compact bone. *Anatom. Rec.* **166**, 247–256.

Suominen, H. (1993) Bone material density and long term exercise. An overview of cross-sectional athlete studies. *Sports Med.* **16**, 316–330.

Tilton, F. E., Degioanni, J. J. and Schneider, V. S. (1980) Long term follow-up of Skylab bone demineralization. *Aviat. Space Environ. Med.* **51**, 1209–1213.

Tram, K. K.-T., Murray, S. S., Lee, D. B. N. and Murray, E. J. B. (1993) PTH-induced osteoblast contraction is mediated by cysteine proteases. *Kidney Int.* **43**, 693–699.

Uy, H. L., Guise, T. A., de la Mata, J. *et al.* (1995) Effects of parathyroid hormone (PTH)-related protein and PTH on osteoclasts and osteoclast precursors *in vivo. Endocrinology* **136**, 3207–3212.

Weinbaum, S., Cowin, S. C. and Zeng, Y. (1994) A model for the excitation of osteocytes by mechanical loading induced bone fluid shear stresses. *J. Biomechan.* **27**, 339–360.

Williams, J. L., Iannotti, J. P., Ham, A., Bleuit, J. and Chen, J. H. (1994) Effects of fluid shear stresses on bone cells. *Biorhealogy* **31**, 163–170.

Wolff, J. (1986) *The Law of Bone Remodeling* (translated by P. Maquet and R. Furlong). Springer Press. Berlin.

15

Mechanical strain-associated nitric oxide production by bone cells

ANDREW A. PITSILLIDES and LANCE E. LANYON

15.1 Mechanically induced adaptive responses in bone

Many observations support the existence of dynamic relationships between the structural load-bearing characteristics of connective tissues and their prevailing mechanical milieu. Indeed, there is much evidence that indicates that once developmental establishment of bone primordia is complete, a primary influence on their shape, structure and mass is derived from their local mechanical environment. The capacity of bone to withstand loads without damage or failure is clearly established and subsequently maintained, at least in part, by such functionally adaptive mechanisms. Roux (1881) and Wolff (1892) both proposed that such 'functional adaptation' was the dominant mechanism by which the organization of bone trabeculae coud provide maximum load-bearing strength with minimum mass. This concept formed the basis of the proposal that necessary functional stimulus for such adaptive responses was derived from loading-induced strains (Frost, 1964).

Such adaptive relationships are responsible for the attainment of structurally appropriate bone mass and architecture (in most locations) at all times, and their effects are clearly evident in the raised bone mass observed with exercise-related increases in load bearing (Smith and Gilligan, 1970; Jones *et al.*, 1997), and the bone loss associated with reduced load bearing (Donaldson *et al.*, 1970). However, on the basis of *in vivo* strain monitoring techniques, it has since become apparent that rather than acting to minimize strain levels, these responses adapt bones so as to control their strain levels during habitual use (Lanyon, 1987). These target strain levels are presumed to be optimal in some respect. Peak strain levels measured on the surface of cortical bone during locomotion, in a wide range of species, show a relatively small variation, with a range of 2000–3000 $\mu\varepsilon$ (Rubin and Lanyon, 1984a).

The mechanism by which these 'target' strain levels are maintained is central to our investigations. It was shown that short daily periods of dynamic load (36 cycles at 0.5 Hz) applied to functionally isolated avian ulnae *in vivo*, producing peak strain levels within the habitual range but with a distribution different from those to which the bone had been architecturally adapted, were sufficient not only to suppress the resorption that would otherwise accompany such functional isolation but also to stimulate increases in bone formation (Lanyon *et al.*, 1982; Rubin and Lanyon, 1984b). These observations were extended by the finding that a single period of such 'novel' loading was an adequate stimulus to convert quiescent periosteal bone surfaces to active bone formation five days later (Pead *et al.*, 1988). This provided a foundation for the consequences of specific, single temporally defined osteogenic loading episodes to be addressed, both *in vivo* and *in vitro*.

Using a range of *in vitro* approaches, much interest has recently focused on the unambiguous identification of the particular parameter, within the mechanical environment, that constitutes the principal influence controlling load bearing-induced structural adaptation *in vivo*. In essence, it is widely accepted that mechanical loading results in three distinct, yet apparently inseparable, sequelae *in vivo*. These are changes in local strain, intralacunar and extracellular matrix-associated fluid flow, and flow-induced streaming or 'stress-generated' electrical potentials.

Recently, Duncan and Turner (1995) suggested that three stages appear to be required in bone's adaptive response to load bearing. These are: (i) the transduction of mechanical events into cellular signals (mechanotransduction); (ii) the intercellular communication of these events, or signals, to establish an assessment of strain distribution; and (iii) the coordination of the consequent (re)modelling events that act in order to alter or maintain the bones' functional competence. However, despite both the sensitivity of these systems to isolated mechanical events and their obvious importance, the cellular mechanisms responsible for their control and regulation remain enigmatic. It is evident that establishing the mechanisms that control each of these stages may provide a cellular basis for preventing disease-associated bone fracture, or indeeed may allow for restoration of bone mass in circumstances, like post-menopausal osteoporosis, where its load-bearing competence would otherwise remain compromised.

15.2 The analogy with endothelium

There is considerable evidence indicating that prostaglandins are produced by bone cells during both the initial mechanotransduction stage and the later loading-engendered osteogenic/anti-resorptive stages (Binderman, Shimshoni and Sömjen, 1984; Yeh and Rodan, 1984). Initially, Jee *et al.* (1987, 1990) demonstrated the osteogenic influence of PGE_2 on bone remodelling *in vivo*. Later, it was found that strain application *in vitro* resulted in increased prostaglandin production by bone cells (Binderman *et al.*, 1988; Murray and Rushton, 1990; Brighton *et al.*, 1991), and that *in vivo* indomethacin treatment modulated loading-induced osteogenesis (Jee *et al.*, 1987; Pead and Lanyon, 1989; Chow and Chambers, 1994). The role of prostaglandins in the early loading-induced responses is also supported by studies indicating that PGI_2 and PGE_2 release is increased during loading of canine cancellous bone cores maintained in short-term superfusion culture (Rawlinson *et al.*, 1991). The functional role for prostaglandins *in vivo* was shown by the fact that indomethacin administration abrogated the acute load-related increases in resident osteoblast and osteocyte glucose 6-phosphate dehydrogenase (G6PD) activity, which are normally associated with their response to dynamic mechanical load application (Skerry *et al.*, 1989; Pead and Lanyon 1989; Dallas *et al.*, 1993; Dodds *et al.*, 1993).

Recently, these findings were extended by more direct evidence indicating that administration of minimal osteogenic response-inducing doses of PGE_2 could, when combined with the application of minimal osteogenic response-inducing loads, produce synergistic effects at the periosteal, but not the endosteal, surfaces (Tang *et al.*, 1997). Therefore, it is apparent that bone cells are capable of producing prostaglandins in response to increases in load-bearing and that this is linked to the consequences of such mechanical stimulation.

In many situations, the production and release of prostaglandins is intimately linked and closely associated with the release of NO. Indeed, it is now well established that endothelial cells contribute to vascular tone control by releasing dilator molecules, such as PGI_2, as well as more elusive molecules such as endothelial-derived hyperpolarizing factor. We now also appreciate that this vasodilatory role is not restricted to these molecules, as it is now apparent that NO is also a potent vasodilator and is, like PGI_2, an excellent inhibitor of platelet aggregation.

These parallels between the functions of NO and PGI_2, as well as others regarding the regulation of the enzymes responsible for their production, namely NOS and COX, are increasingly becoming more extensive. Indeed, recent observations indicate that laminar shear stress applied to endothelial cells *in vitro* produces rapid enhancement of PGI_2 release (Frangos *et al.*, 1985; Hecker *et al.*, 1993), which is apparently accompanied by the release of NO (Kuchan and Frangos, 1994). This led us to investigate the possibility that NO release may also be involved in bones' mechanoadaptive responses (Pitsillides *et al.*, 1995a, b).

15.3 Analogies between the development of neuronal long-term potentiation/depression and the 'strain memory' concept

In addition to being involved in strain transduction, NO could contribute to consequent cell–cell communication. In the nervous system, a mechanism that is dependent on the production of NO has been proposed to explain both long-term potentiation and long-term depression of signalling (Garthwaite, Charles and Chess-Williams, 1988; Bohme *et al.*, 1991; Dawson and Snyder, 1994). This is considered to be responsible for imparting a 'plasticity' on the magnitude of transmitted signals; for this reason it is believed that such a mechanism is important for the generation of 'memory' in nervous tissue. This paradigm is attractive when it is considered in bone tissue, as it provides clear analogies with the mechanistic prerequisites of the strain-sensitive adaptive responses that maintain functionally appropriate bone mass and architecture.

A communicative function is clearly essential in order to establish a collective assessment of strain distribution in bone. Further, the recognition events that either maintian bones' status quo or coordinate any osteogenic/anti-resorptive events which are necessary to attain functional load-bearing competence, require that the cells responsible for perceiving alterations in strain are previously attuned to some optimum 'target strain'. This has led to the development of the 'strain memory' concept, which has been used to describe the means by which resident bone cells recognize only novel magnitudes or distributions of strain. It is clear that plasticity of signalling, or an ability to alter the strain-sensitive characteristics of the resident bone cells, would be beneficial in such a system. Therefore, it is an attractive possibility that such locally controlled 'signalling plasticity' may also exist within resident bone cell networks, and that NO, via a mechanism similar to that which exists in the nervous system, may be involved in its control. Further, this may, if substantiated, explain why cells of the osteoblastic lineage maintain an inherent 'neuronal-like' spatial connectivity.

Coupled with the endothelial paradigm involving a role for NO and PGI_2 in the transduction of mechanical events into cellular signals, and their proposed role in intercellular communication, this clearly establishes NO as an obvious candidate molecule to contribute to the coordination of events responsible for maintaining the structural load-bearing competence of bone.

15.4 Do mechanical stimuli result in NO production by bone cells?

Many studies have shown that NO release can be stimulated in bone cells, and several of these have addressed their response to mechanical stimuli.

Initially, in order to establish whether bone cells were capable of producing NO, long-term (> 8 h) cytokine-induced increases in NO release were shown using primary rat osteoblast-like cells, UMR-106 (Löwik et al., 1994) and the MC3T3-E1 clonal cell line (Damoulis and Hauschka, 1994). Later, using [^{3}H]thymidine incorporation and RT-PCR analysis of human osteoblast-like cells isolated from orthopaedic surgical specimens, it was concluded that such cytokine-induced transcriptional control of iNOS-mediated NO release constitutes a suppressive regulatory factor of osteoblastic cell proliferation. RT-PCR analysis showed that ROS 17/2.8 cells express iNOS and at least one cNOS isoform without cytokine pre-treatment and that increases in proliferation were associated with increased levels of NO release, while NOS inhibitors dose-dependently decreased proliferation. Although these studies provide conflicting data concerning NO's role in osteoblast proliferation, they clearly show that bone cells are capable of NO release, and that alterations in NO production can be transcriptionally controlled, with measurable increases evident about 6–8 h after cytokine treatment (Chapters 10 and 11).

15.4.1 Mechanical loading of bone in organ culture

In order to address our hypothesis that bone cell-derived NO is released in response to mechanical loading-induced strains, we initially examined whether NO release from bone organ cultures was influenced by loads that created strains of physiological magnitudes. Using cultured canine cancellous bone cores (marrow removed) and chemiluminescent assessment of nitrite concentration in single passage super-fusate, we found that rates of NO release were (i) increased during a period that encompassed loading; (ii) reached mean rates significantly higher than in controls after 15 min; and (iii) showed no further increases in the subsequent 30 min. The timing of these changes was similar to those previously described for PGI_2 and PGE_2 (Rawlinson *et al.*, 1991), indicating that there were rapid loading-induced increases in NO release. NO decreased to control levels promptly upon withdrawal of the loading stimulus.

To establish whether such NO release was solely a feature of trabecular bone, we examined the effect of load on cortical bone *in vitro* and found that rat ulnar (cartilaginous ends and marrow removed) explants produced significant and, in this case, strain magnitude-related increases in NO release (Pitsillides *et al.*, 1995b) (Figure 15.1). The enzymatic source of these load-induced increases in NO release was confirmed by their reduction in the presence of the NOS inhibitors L-NAME and L-N^5-(1-iminoethyl)ornithine (L-NIO).

These studies demonstrated clearly that NO release was stimulated rapidly in response to dymanic loads. However, at this stage it was not known whether loading might also induce longer-term increases in NO release. Therefore, we examined NO release from rat caudal vertebrae, cultured as described by Bourrin and co-workers (1994), and found that loads (31 N) engendering 2200 µε (1 Hz, 10 min) induced significant short-term increases in NO release. Nevertheless, although such

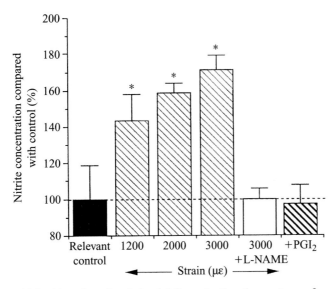

Figure 15.1. Alterations in nitrite (µM) production (percentage of respective contralateral control, mean ± SEM) by rat ulnae induced by (i) different levels of mechanical strain (1200–3000 µε) in the absence of L-NAME, (ii) mechanical strain (3000 µε) in the presence of L-NAME (100 µM) and (iii) 1 mM prostacyclin ($n = 3$ experiments in each case). *denotes significance at a level of $p < 0.05$.

transient increases in NO release were evident during each of four separate periods of load (24 h apart), increased rates of NO release were not apparent over any of the ensuing 24-h periods (Figure 15.2). This is consistent with a rapid stimulation of a non-permanent loading-induced increase in the rate of NO production. The transient nature of these increases, as well as their prompt deactivation upon removal of mechanical loads, suggests the involvement of a cNOS, and not iNOS, isoform in these responses.

15.4.2 Response of bone cells in monolayer culture

Several studies have investigated the possibility that monolayer cultures of bone cells respond to mechanical stimuli by increasing their production of NO and other autocoids. These studies can, for discussion purposes, be subdivided on the basis that they examine the response either to the application of mechanical strain or to fluid flow. The notion that load-induced fluid flow plays a role in the control of bone (re)modelling has been considered by many (Gross and Williams, 1982; Pollack *et al.*, 1984; Cowin and Sadegh, 1991; Jones and Bingmann, 1992; Lanyon, 1992; Weinbaum, Cowin and Zeng, 1994). *In vivo* observations have shown that bone mass increases in the skull and mandible, is not changed in the fore limbs and decreases in the hind limbs of rats subjected to several weeks of tail suspension (Roer and Dillaman, 1990). Similar changes are evident in humans subjected to head-down tilt bedrest, suggesting that cephalic fluid shift and the resultant increases in flow rates, and shear strains that they engender, directly increase bone mass in the skull (Arnaud *et al.*, 1988), while decreases in fluid

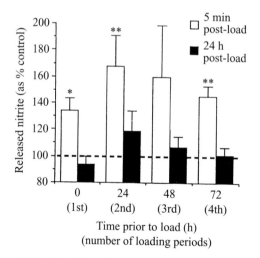

Figure 15.2. The effect of repeated applications (four) of mechanical load (over a period of 72 h) on the concentration of released nitrite (expressed as percentage of control; mean $\pm$ SEM) from rat vertebrae ($n = 6$). Percentage increases over control values at both 5 min and 24 h after each load application are indicated. * and ** denote significance at a level of $p < 0.05$ and $p < 0.025$, respectively.

flow in hind limbs may be responsible for bone loss (Dillaman *et al.*, 1991; see also Chapters 13 and 14).

Along these lines, it has been shown that rat calvarial-derived osteoblast-like cells responded dose dependently to theoretically predicted rates of laminar fluid flow by rapid increase in PGE$_2$ release, which were sustainable (for at least 8 h) and accompanied by increased intracellular inositol triphosphate (IP$_3$) levels. Further, based on their partial inhibition by indomethacin, it was suggested that these responses were at least partly dependent on flow-induced prostaglandin production (Reich and Frangos, 1991). These findings have recently been extended by those of Ajubi and co-workers (1996) in which osteoblasts, osteocytes and periosteal fibroblasts derived from fetal chick calvariae all showed increased PGI$_2$ and PGE$_2$ release in response to the application of pulsatile fluid flow (0.5 ± 0.02 Pa, 5 Hz). Their results suggest that osteocytes produce the most marked increases in PGI$_2$ and PGE$_2$ release, and that osteocytic PGE$_2$ release rates apparently decline rapidly during the 1 h flow period, while rates of PGI$_2$ release decline less obviously.

Interestingly, using similar magnitudes and duration (1 h) of fluid flow, Klein-Nulend and co-workers (1995a) showed that in a period of 1 h after the cessation of such pulsatile fluid flow (0.5 ± 0.02 Pa, 5 Hz) there were significant increases in the sustained rates of release of PGE$_2$, but not PGI$_2$, from osteocytes but not from osteoblasts or periosteal fibroblasts. On this basis, it was proposed that post-flow increases in osteocyte PGE$_2$ release may reflect its proposed role in 'strain memory'. However, it is possible that this might reflect the relative contribution of different prostaglandins to early flow-induced events, suggesting that PGI$_2$, but not PGE$_2$, has a role in osteocyte flow perception; alternatively, if the osteocyte-selective sustainable increase in post-load PGE$_2$, but not PGI$_2$, release is reproduced *in vivo*, this may reflect a role for PGE$_2$ in some other post-loading event.

A few studies have recently addressed the possibility that NO may also be involved in bone cell responses to mechanical stimuli. Indeed, calvaria-derived chick osteocytes, but not periosteal fibroblasts, appear to respond to the application of pulsating fluid flow (0.5 ± 0.02 Pa, 5 Hz, 0.4 Pa/s) with rapid elevation in NO and PGE$_2$ release rates, both of which are inhibited by the NOS inhibitor L-NMMA (Klein-Nulend *et al.*, 1995b). Similarly, increased laminar fluid flow (6 dyne/cm^2) also results in a dexamethasone-insensitive stimulation in NO release from osteoblast-like cells, the rate of which was sustained during 12 h of continued flow (Johnson *et al.*, 1996). Interestingly, it has been proposed that flow-related NO (and PGI$_2$) release from human umbilical vein endothelial cells has two distinct components; one which is induced by the onset (or burst) of flow, and a second stimulated, thereafter, by steady rates of flow (Frangos *et al.*, 1985; Kuchan and Frangos, 1994). Briefly, the application of impulse-like increases in flow stimulate only G-protein-dependent bursts in NO release. In contrast, ramped increases in flow fail to stimulate bursts in NO release but do yield sustained NO release. Step-wise increases in flow, which have both rapid and steady flow components, stimulate both pathways (Frangos, Huang and Clark, 1996; see also Chapter 14). Therefore, care should be taken in drawing conclusions from such studies in bone cells, as it is clear that pulsatile fluid flow-induced increases in the rate of NO (and PGI_2) release from osteoblasts and osteocytes may reflect their response to the pulsatile nature of the flow to which they are exposed, and not necessarily to flow itself.

We have found that increased NO release is also evident in monolayer cultures of osteoblast-like cells and embryonic chick osteocytes subjected to physiological levels of mechanical strain. In both these cells of the osteoblast lineage, we found that NO release was rapidly stimulated upon application of mechanical strain (within minutes), and that this increased rate of NO release was non-permanent, returning to basal levels on cessation of strain application. Indeed, preliminary evidence indicates that an extension of the loading period prolongs these elevated rates of NO release (unpublished observations).

Together, these studies suggest that increases in NO release stimulated by both flow and mechanical strain involve the activation of a constitutively expressed NOS isoform. It is evident that either interstitial flow or strain, or both (or indeed one via the agency of the other), may mediate skeletal remodelling in response to changes in mechanical loading. The view that altered rates of fluid flow form the stimulus that initiates bone's adaptive resposes is not novel (Salzstein *et al.*, 1987; Salzstein and Pollack, 1987; Kufahl and Saha, 1990; Turner, Forwood and Otter, 1994). It is based on the notion that bones behave much like relatively stiff fluid-filled sponges, and that when they are exposed to loading, which results in a strain gradient, fluid will be forced from the area of greatest compression to where it is least.

Consistent with this notion of a flow-induced stimulation of osteogenesis, it was found that the application of 4-point bending loads (of increasing frequency) to rat tibiae for 15 days resulted in frequency-related increases in endocortical bone formation rate (Turner *et al.*, 1994). Loading frequency also increased stress-generated potentials, measured in similar bones *ex vivo*, suggesting that increases in interstitial flow may directly affect the stimulus for bone formation. However, these conclusions do not explain the observed consequences of increased load-bearing *in vivo*. Unless the well-established coordination of functionally associated loading-induced adaptive (re)modelling in bone is geared to achieve some 'target rate of fluid-flow' in bone, then these findings provide a fragmentary understanding of the mechanisms by which bones' load-bearing competence, with its encumbant require-ment for 'optimum' strains, is established and maintained.

It is, however, possible that the mechanical strain-related stimulus has multiple origins and has as a component the rate of fluid flow, and that this facilitates subsequent alterations in (re)modelling. Nevertheless, restoration of 'target' strains appears to be, in practical terms, the ultimate aim of these events *in vivo*, and it is apparent that, *in vitro*, where cells are removed from their normal milieu such specific features of their responsiveness may, to some extent, become compromised.

15.5 How are load-related NO and prostaglandin production related?

A key question raised by these initial findings was whether this rapid production and release of NO was induced by or was necessary to stimulate the previously described load-induced increase in prostaglandin production. Many investigations suggest that both NO- and PGI_2-generating mechanisms are stimulated in a coordinated manner via well-defined independent pathways (Shrör *et al.*, 1991) and that dynamic interplay exists between prostaglandin mediated cAMP production and cNOS-mediated stimulation of cGMP production (Salvemini *et al.*, 1993; Vane *et al.*, 1994). This is complicated by conflicting observations that have suggested that NO appears to either stimulate or inhibit prostaglandin synthesis (Keen, Pickering and Hunt, 1990; Salvemini, Currie and Hollace, 1996) and that inhibitors of NOS activity are capable of either decreasing or increasing prostaglandin production (Keen *et al.*, 1990; Davidge *et al.*, 1995). Therefore, the relationship between the production of these mediators is by no means clear.

This apparent lack of clarity is also evident in bone cell responses to mechanical stimuli. Using rat ulnae in organ culture and long bone-derived osteoblast-like cells, we have found no alterations in the rate of NO release either 15 min or 8 h after addition of exogenous PGI_2. However, we also found (unpublished) that both indomethacin and 15-hydroperoxyeicosatetraenoic acid (a selective PGI_2 synthase inhibitor (Mayer *et al.*, 1986)) prevented load-induced NO release (Pitsillides *et al.*, 1995b), suggesting that, in culture at least, load-related stimulation of NO release is reliant upon a functional PGI_2-generating system, while being independent of a direct effect of PGI_2 itself. It has also been shown (Klein-Nulend *et al.*, 1995b) that a non-selective NOS inhibitor, L-NMMA, blocked pulsating fluid flow-induced increase in both NO and PGE_2 release. This emphasizes the complexity of these relationships and highlights the need for further studies to establish the manner by which these autocoids interact in bone.

One means by which these questions may be simplified is by addressing them *in situ*, where resident bone cells may maintain behavioural characteristics that are related to their anatomical location. A number of studies have shown that glucose 6-phosphate dehydrogenase (G6PD) activity in resident osteoblasts and osteocytes increases in a strain magnitude-dependent manner immediately following the application of osteogenic loads *in vivo*; it is apparent that these changes may reflect the consequent alterations in (re)modelling which occur some time later (Dallas *et al.*, 1993; Dodds *et al.*, 1993). Such increases in G6PD activity are reproduced in organ culture and are also stimulated dose dependently by exogenous prostaglandins (Rawlinson *et al.*, 1993), including PGI_2, which appears to be produced by osteocytes and osteoblasts, and PGE_2, produced in osteoblasts alone (Rawlinson *et al.*, 1991). Therefore, it is possible that loading-induced increases in osteocyte-derived NO release may be linked, either directly or indirectly, via intimately coupled PGI_2 production to strain-related changes in G6PD activity, suggesting that NO release is an integral component of such adaptive responses. Along these lines, a study by Zaman *et al.* (1997) showed that while both exogenous PGI_2 and PGE_2 produced increases in osteoblast-like cell G6PD activity, PGI_2, but not PGE_2, stimulated similar transcript-selective increases in mRNA for IGF-II, but not IGF-I, as those induced by mechanical strain application.

15.6 Do non-load-bearing bones release NO in response to loading?

In contrast to the strain magnitude-related NO release evident in loaded long bones in culture, loading of cultured rat calvariae (1 Hz for 10 min, peak principal compressive strains of either 100 or 1000 $\mu\varepsilon$) to engender strains greater than those measured *in vivo* (Rawlinson *et al.*, 1995) do not produce significant increase in NO release. This insensitivity of 'non-load bearing' calvariae *in vitro* agrees with our earlier studies, which indicated that calvarially derived osteoblast-like cells and resident osteoblasts and osteocytes in cultured calvarial bones failed to show any loading-related increases in G6PD activity (Rawlinson *et al.*, 1995). Therefore, it is tempting to speculate that these responses are related to the distinct 'protective' role of calvarial bones and the 'weight-bearing' role of long bones. The structural competence of calvariae, but not long bones, is in excess of their habitual load-bearing demands and, therefore, these bones may achieve their bone mass and architecture by different mechanisms. This may also be of relevance when considering how osteoblast-like cells derived from calvariae respond to mechanical stimulation *in vitro*.

15.7 Which bone cells are responsible for NO production?

There is already much evidence regarding the ability of bone cells, partucularly osteoblasts and osteoclasts, to both respond to and produce NO, and this will be dealt with, in great detail, by others in this volume. Our studies indicate that rat long bone-derived osteoblast-like cells are capable of producing rapid increases in NO release in response to strains of physiological magnitude *in vitro* (Pitsillides *et al.*, 1995b); while we have shown that similar loading regimens also stimulate both osteoblast proliferation and differentiation (Cheng *et al.*, 1994, 1996), we have not, to date, provided information regarding the precise cellular source of strain-induced NO production in intact bones.

More recently, comparing strain-induced NO release from osteoblast-like cells derived from calvariae and femurs, we found that both produced significant increases in nitrite accumulation, indicating similarities in their NO-related responsiveness to mechanical strain. As intact calvariae in organ culture showed no load-related increases in NO release (G. Zaman, R. F. L. Suswillo, M. Z. Cheng *et al.*, unpublished data), these results appear paradoxical. Therefore, it is logical to assume that osteoblasts (and osteocytes) in intact calvariae are relatively insensitive to direct strain, and that the isolation of osteoblast-like cells from these bones increases their exposure to a component, or derivative, of load from which they are protected *in situ*. Alternatively, their sensitivity might be increased as a result of isolation and culture. Further, based on their failure to show strain-related increases in G6PD activity in culture (Rawlinson *et al.*, 1995), it is also clear that this is unrelated to their strain-induced NO release.

15.7.1 *Strain-related NO production by osteocytes*

We hypothesize that a communicating network of osteocytes has an essential role in bones' response to load bearing and that by processing mechanically related information they collectively influence (re)modelling events. This hypothesis is not original; however, it has recently become increasingly amenable to investigation. Its substantiation requires the direct demonstration that osteocytes exhibit behavioural changes that are related, obligatorily, to the strain-related control of mechanically adaptive architectural changes in (re)modelling. Using immunomagnetically isolated osteocytes (van der Plaas and Nijweide, 1992) from 18 day old embryonic chick tibiotarsi (using MAb 7.3(5); kind gift from Prof. P. J. Nijweide), we showed that these cells exhibited significant increases in NO release following strain application. It is apparent that cells at this distinct 'end-stage' of osteoblast differentiation are capable of rapid strain-induced increases in NO release (Pitsillides *et al.*, 1995c). However, the degree to which osteocytic differentiation controls the magnitude of this response is unknown.

To address this, we used osteoblast-like cells and osteocytes both derived from embryonic chick long bones. We found that in response to similar mechanical strain levels, osteocytes produced greater load-specific NO release than osteoblast-like cells; with the latter producing 2.40 ± 0.10 pMNO/h per cell and osteocytes producing enhanced rates of release of 8.32 ± 2.40 pMNO/h per cell (Pitsillides *et al.*, 1997). This suggests that strain-related NO release within intact bones may be predominantly osteocytic. As it is well established that osteocytes are the most prominent cell type in bone, these findings suggest that osteocytes, and not osteoblasts, constitute the main source of bone cell strain-related NO release.

15.7.2 *Which isoform of NOS is expressed by bone cells?*

NO can be generated by three distinct NOS isofoms (Chapter 1). Based on the potential for transcriptional and post-translational activation of these isoforms, it is apparent from the rapidity of load-induced increases in NO release that these are mediated by a cNOS, and not iNOS, isoform. Using RT-PCR analysis, it has been shown that cultured osteoblast-like cells express all three isoforms: iNOS (Ralston *et al.*, 1994; Pitsillides *et al.*, 1995b; Riancho *et al.*, 1995), eNOS (Riancho *et al.*, 1995) and nNOS (Pitsillides *et al.*, 1995b). Such RT-PCR analyses fail, however, to provide clear quantitative results concerning relative mRNA expression and, while useful in detecting rare transcripts, the expression patterns depend on primer amplification efficiencies of the respective mRNA. Therefore, NOS mRNA expression and distribution in bone is not established.

Northern blot hybridization of total RNA from fresh rat ulnae and calvariae

(Chomczynski and Saatchi, 1987) indicated that the apparent PCR-based multiplicity of NOS gene expression by bone cells is not observed. Using probe sequences for nNOS (Bredt *et al.*, 1991), iNOS (Nunokawa, Ishida and Tanaka, 1993) and eNOS (Nudel *et al.*, 1983), neither nNOS nor iNOS transcripts were detected in RNA from ulnae, calvariae or long bone osteoblast-like cells; in contrast, eNOS transcripts were detected in RNA from all these sources (G. Zaman *et al.*, unpublished data).

Immunocytochemistry also showed that eNOS was most extensively expressed by cells of the osteoblast lineage. iNOS labelling was very weak in both osteoblasts and osteocytes in rat calvariae and ulnae, and relatively weak nNOS labelling was observed only in calvarial osteocytes. In contrast, eNOS labelling was very prominent in mid-cortical osteocytes in ulnae. Osteoblasts in both ulnae and calvariae showed less clear eNOS staining, while eNOS-positive osteocytes are absent in calvariae. Therefore, osteocyte eNOS may contribute to their strain-related NO production in long bones, and the lack of osteocyte eNOS in calvariae may reflect either their proposed lack of mechanical responsiveness or that pathways involved in their (re)modelling control are eNOS independent.

However, despite the relative absence of detectable eNOS protein in these bones, our Northern blot hybridization results confirm eNOS mRNA in calvariae. Paradoxically, this suggest that eNOS mRNA translation in calvariae may be limited and may support the notion that calvarial osteocytes are not exposed to strain levels that stimulate eNOS mRNA translation. As calvariae-derived osteoblast-like cells do show increased NO release in response to strain, this suggests that up-regulation of NOS protein, possibly eNOS, might occur in cultured calvarially derived cells. Regardless, it is clear that the predominant isoform of NOS expressed by cells of the osteoblast lineage is eNOS, and that this is expressed markedly by osteocytes within bone.

15.7.3 Which bone cells are affected by NOS inhibition in vivo?

Recently, it has been observed that both mechanically induced osteogensis in rat tail vertebrae and four-point bending-induced osteogenic responses in rat tibiae can be abrogated by intraperitoneal L-NMMA (Fox, Chambers and Chow, 1996) or oral L-NAME, respectively (Turner *et al.*, 1996). This suggests that NOS inhibitors block loading-induced changes while they fail to affect normal bone remodelling. We have shown that long-term L-NAME administration, at concentrations shown to produce increases in blood pressure, does not produce any marked changes in osteoblast G6PD activity. This suggests that basal levels of osteoblastic G6PD activity may reflect normal bone modelling, which is not necessarily directly linked to bone cell strain-related NO production but is predominantly regulated by NO-independent factors associated with growth. In contrast, osteocytes in the ulnar mid-cortex of L-NAME-treated rats showed decreases in G6PD activity, suggesting that NO may be responsible for maintaining osteocyte, but no osteoblast, G6PD activity (A. A. Pitsillides, G. Zaman, S. C. F. Rawlinson *et al.*, unpublishing data). This may indicate that osteocytic G6PD activity is related to, or perhaps controlled by, endogenous levels of osteocyte NO production. Therefore, transient local decreases in osteocyte G6PD activity or simply the blockade of strain-induced increases in osteocyte G6PD activity, which are normally associated with strain application, may be sufficient to nullify only those osteogenic responses induced directly by such novel strains. This is circumstantial evidence suggesting that osteocytic responses to strain are to some extent dependent on their G6PD activity, and that NOS inhibition-induced loss of load-related osteogenesis may rely on the depression of osteocytic, but not osteoblastic, G6PD activity. Alternatively, it is possible that basal levels of osteocytic, but not osteoblastic, G6PD activity are controlled by local NO production. Therefore, both G6PD activity and osteocyte NO production may be involved in osteocytic perception of changes in load bearing.

These results also raise the possibility that osteocyte- (and perhaps osteoblast-) derived, eNOS-mediated strain-induced NO production may influence local blood vessel tone. Changes in load-bearing, producing local strains with either different magnitude or different distribution from that to which the bone is architecturally adapted, will induce spatially appropriate increases in eNOS-derived NO release. These increases may act to modulate bone formation and resorption directly or may create the necessary local conditions required for functionally desirable (re)modelling events, via an indirect coherent influence on blood flow. This is consistent with the well-established paradigm in which fluid flow-induced endothelial cell NO release contributes to vascular tone. It is tempting to speculate that our results identify a fundamental, and potentially influential, extension to the sphere of influence of this paradigm. The results could be interpreted to indicate the effects of mechanical strain, or one of its immediate derivatives in bone, could be measured by the specific distribution and quantity of osteocyte-derived NO, and that NO's long-term osteogenic contribution could be mediated by indirect regulation of local blood flow. Therefore, if NO derived by such a mechanism does not affect bone formation or resorption directly, it remains possible that it may act as a facilitator of these responses.

15.7.4 How is cNOS activity regulated by ion channels in bone cells?

Endothelial cells lack voltage-gated calcium channels (Davies, 1995). This finding may be relevant to the situation in bone, where osteoblasts, but not osteocytes, appear to posses such nifedipine-sensitive voltage-gated calcium channel activities (Rawlinson *et al.*, 1996). This is a clear similarity between osteocytes and endothelial cells with respect to ion channel activity and is supported by findings which indicate that osteocytes, as well as endothelial cells (and osteoblasts), possess stretch-shear (gadolinium-sensitive) cation channels (Takeda, Schini and Stoeckel, 1987; Olesen, Clapham and Davies, 1988; Kamioka *et al.*, 1995; Rawlinson *et al.*, 1996). Therefore, osteocyte maturation may involve their selective maintenance of endothelial-like channel activities, the concurrent loss of osteoblast-specific channel-related character and increased eNOS expression.

15.8 Conclusions

Rapid load-induced increases in NO release by cells of the osteoblast lineage are likely to be an important influence in adaptive bone (re)modelling. Our findings have provided evidence that these loading-induced responses are evident in isolated bone cells, that in whole bones this NO release may be predominantly osteocytic in origin, that such increases are mediated by post-translational increases in eNOS activity and that this is intimately linked to prostanoid production. These findings appear to be consistent with the well-established paradigm in which fluid flow-induced endothelial cell NO production contributes to vascular tone, and it is tempting to speculate that our results suggest that osteocyte NO release is similarly involved in bones's response to its mechanical environment. This possibility represents a fundamental, and potentially influential, extension to the sphere of influence of this paradigm.

Furthermore, recent evidence using brain slices from eNOS knock-out mice have suggested that long-term potentiation, which is often considered to be a cellular correlate of learning, requires NO synthesized by eNOS in post-synaptic cells as a retrograde messenger (Wilson *et al.*, 1997). Such potentiation, as well as depression, of signalling has for some time been attributed solely to the nNOS isoform, and for this reason we proposed such a role for bone cell nNOS, based on our RT-PCR findings (Pitsillides *et al.*, 1995b). These novel findings, however, extend eNOS' functions to include the control of such 'signalling plasticity', and it remains possible that load-related, eNOS-mediated, bone cell NO release may alter bone cell network characteristics in a manner similar to that which exists in the nervous system and that such a mechanism is responsible for what has become known as 'strain-memory'.

Recently, it was shown that an NO donor was capable of attenuating ovariectomy-induced bone loss in rats and that some of oestrogen's beneficial effects on bone appear to be mediated by NO (Wimalawansa *et al.*, 1996). It is also clear that modulating loading-associated NO production by bone cells may provide a preventative or restorative basis for facilitating architecturally appropriate increases in bone mass in situations (like postmenopausal osteoporosis) where bones' load-bearing competence would otherwise remain compromised.

Acknowledgements

We thank Prof. S. Moncada, Dr R. G. Knowles and particularly Dr Angela Deakin and Mr Neale Foxwell (Pharmacology Department), Wellcome Research Laboratories (Beckenham, UK) who provided the technical facilities to measure nitrite concentration. We also thank Prof. P. J. Nijweide (University of Leiden, the Netherlands) for providing antibody MAb 7.3(5), Dr Shu-Fang Liu (Royal Brompton Hospital, London, UK) for iNOS primers. The authors would also like to thank all the members of the Bone Unit at the Royal Veterinary College (particularly Rosemary Suscuillo, Simon Rawlinson, Gul Zaman, Ming Zioou Cheng and John

Mosley) for their help in completing this work. This work was funded by the Biotechnology and Biological Sciences Research Council (UK, Grant No.: 48/ A1071), The Wellcome Trust, The Arthritis and Rheumatism Council and The Medical Research Council.

References

Ajubi, N. E., Klein-Nulend, J., Nijweide, P. J., Vrijheidlammers, T., Alblas, M. J. and Berger, E. H. (1996) Pulsating fluid-flow increases prostaglandin production by cultured chicken osteocytes – a cytoskeleton-dependent process. *Biochem. Biophys. Res. Commun.* **255**, 62–68.

Arnaud, S. B., Powell, M., Vernikos-Danellis, J. and Buchanan, P. (1988) Bone mineral and body composition after 30 day head down tilt bed rest. *J. Bone Min. Res.* **3**, S119.

Binderman, I., Shimshoni, Z. and Sömjen, D. (1984) Biochemical pathways involved in the translation of physical stimulus into biochemical message. *Calcif. Tiss. Int.* **36**, S82–S85.

Binderman, I., Zor, U., Kaye, A. M., Shimshoni, Z., Harell, A. and Sömjen, D. (1988) Transduction of mechanical force into biochemical events in bone cells may involve activation of phospholipase A_2. *Calcif. Tiss. Int.* **42**, 261–266.

Bohme, G. A., Bon, C., Stutzmann, J.-M., Doble, A. and Blanchard, J.-C. (1991) Possible involvement of NO in long-term potentiation. *Eur. J. Pharmacol.* **199**, 379–381.

Bourrin, S., Suswillo, R. F. L. and Lanyon, L. E. (1994) Cancellous bone cells response to artificially engendered dynamic strains *in vitro* using the rat tail vertebra in organ culture. *J. Bone Min. Res.* **9** (Suppl. 1), S255.

Bredt, D. S., Hwang, P. M., Glatt, C. E., Lowenstein, C., Reed, R. R. and Snyder, S. H. (1991) Cloned and expressed nitric oxide synthase structurally resembles cytochrome P-450 reductase. *Nature* **351**, 714–718.

Brighton, C. T., Strafford, B., Gross, S. B., Leatherwood, D., Williams, J. L. and Pollack, S. R. (1991) Proliferative and synthetic response of isolated calvarial bone cells of rats to cyclical biaxial mechanical strain. *J. Bone Joint Surg.* **73A**, 320–331.

Cheng, M. Z., Zaman, G. and Lanyon, L. E. (1994) Estrogen enhances the stimulation of bone collagen synthesis by loading and exogenous prostacyclin, but not prostaglandin E_2, in organ cultures of rat ulnae. *J. Bone Min. Res.* **9**, 805–816.

Cheng, M. Z., Zaman, G., Rawlinson, S. C. F., Suswillo, R. F. L. and Lanyon, L. E. (1996) Mechanical loading and sex hormone interaction in organ cultures of rat ulnae. *J. Bone Min. Res.* **11**, 502–511.

Chomczynski, P. and Saachi, N. (1987) Single step method of RNA isolation by acid quanidinium thiocyanate phenol chloroform extraction. *Anal. Biochem.* **162**, 156–159.

Chow, J. W. and Chambers, T. J. (1994) Indomethacin has distinct early and late actions on bone formation induced by mechanical stimulation. *Am. J. Physiol.* **267**, E287–292.

Cowin, S. C. and Sadegh, A. M. (1991) Noninteracting modes of stress, strain and energy in anisotropic hard tissues. *J. Biomech.* **24**, 859–867.

Dallas, S. L., Zaman, G., Pead, M. J. and Lanyon, L. E. (1993) Early strain-related changes in cultured embryonic chick tibiotarsi parallel those associated with adaptive modeling *in vivo*. *J. Bone Min. Res.* **8**, 251–259.

Damoulis, P. D. and Hauschka, P. V. (1994) Cytokines induce nitric oxide production in mouse osteoblasts. *Biochem. Biophys. Res. Commun.* **201**, 924–931.

Davidge, S. T., Baker, P. N., McLoughlin, M. K. and Roberts, J. M. (1995) Nitric oxide produced by endothelial cells increases production of eicosanoids through activation of prostaglandin H synthase. *Circ. Res.* **77**, 274–283.

Davies, P. F. (1995) Flow-mediated endothelial mechanotransduction. *Physiol. Rev.* **75**, 519–560.

Dawson, T. M. and Snyder, S. H. (1994) Gases as biological messengers: nitric oxide and carbon monoxide in the brain. *J. Neurosci.* **14**, 5147–5159.

Dillaman, R. M., Roer, R. D. and Gay, D. M. (1991) Fluid movement in bone: theorectical and empirical. *J. Biomech.* **24**(Suppl. 1), 163–177.

Dodds, R. A., Ali, N., Pead, M. J. and Lanyon, L. E. (1993) Early loading-related changes in the activity of G6PD and ALP in osteocytes and periosteal osteoblasts in rat fibulae *in vivo. J. Bone Min. Res.* **8**, 261–267.

Donaldson, C. L., Hulley, S. B. Vofel, J., Hattner, R. S., Bayers, J. H. and McMillan, D. E. (1970) Effect of prolonged bed rest on bone mineral. *Metabolism* **19**, 1071–1084.

Duncan, R. L. and Turner, C. H. (1995) Mechanotransduction and the functional response of bone to mechanical strain. *Calcif. Tiss. Int.* **57**, 344–358.

Fox, S. W., Chambers, T. J. and Chow, J. W. M. (1996) Nitric oxide is an early mediator of the increase in bone formation by mechanical stimulation. *Am. J. Physiol.* **270**, E955–E960.

Frangos, J. A., Eskin, S. G., McIntire, L. and Ives, C. L. (1985) Flow effects on prostacyclin production by cultured human endothelial cells. *Science* **227**, 1477–1479.

Frangos, J. A., Huang, T. and Clark, C. B. (1996) Steady shear and step changes in shear stimulate endothelium via independent mechanisms: superposition of transient and sustained NO production. *Biochem. Biophys. Res. Commun.* **224**, 660–665.

Frost, H. M. (1964) *Laws of Bone Structure*. Charles C. Thomas, Springfield, IL.

Garthwaite, J., Charles, S. L. and Chess-Williams, R. (1988) Endothelium-derived relaxing factor release on activation of NMDA receptors suggests role as intercellular messenger in the brain. *Nature* **336**, 385–387.

Gross, D. and Williams, W. S. (1982) Streaming potentials and the electromechanical response of physiologically moist bones. *J. Biomech.* **15**, 277–295.

Hecker, M., Mulsch A., Bassenge, E. and Busse, R. (1993) Vasoconstriction and increased flow – principle mechamisms of shear stress-dependent endothelial autocoid release. *Am. J. Physiol.* **265**, H828–H833.

Jee, W. S. S., Ueno, K., Kimmel, D. B., Woodbury, D. M., Price, P. and Woodbury, L. A. (1987) The role of bone cells in increasing metaphyseal hard tissue in rapidly growing rats treated with prostaglandin E_2. *Bone* **8**, 171–178.

Jee, W. S. S., Mori, S., Li, X. I. and Chan, S. (1990) Prostaglandin E_2 enhances cortical bone mass and activates intracortical remodelling in intact and ovariectomised female rats. *Bone* **11**, 253–266.

Johnson, D. L., McAllister, T. N. and Frangos, J. A. (1996) Fluid-flow stimulates rapid and continuous release of nitric oxide in osteoblasts. *Am. J. Physiol.* **271**, E205–E208.

Jones, D. B. and Bingmann, D. (1992) How do osteoblasts respond to mechanical stimulation. *Cells Mater.* **1**, 329–340.

Jones, H. H., Priest, J. D. and Hayes, W. C. (1977) Humeral hypertrophy in response to exercise. *J. Bone Joint Surg.* **59A**, 204–208.

Kamioka, M. H., Miki, Y., Sumitani, K., Tagami, K., Hosoi, K. and Kamata, T. (1995) *Biochem. Biophys. Res. Commun.* **212**, 692–696.

Keen, M., Pickering, S. and Hunt, J. A. (1990) Modulation of the bradykinin-stimulated release of prostacyclin from endothelial cells. *Br. J. Pharmacol.* **101**, 534P.

Klein-Nulend, J., van der Plaas, A., Semeins, C. M. *et al.* (1995a) Sensitivity of osteocytes to biomechanical stress *in vitro. FASEB J.* **9**, 441–445.

Klein-Nulend, J., Semeins, C. M., Ajubi, N. E., Nijweide, P. J. and Berger, E. H. (1995b) Pulsating fluid flow increases nitric oxide (NO) synthesis by osteocytes but not periosteal fibroblasts – correlation with prostaglandin up-regulation. *Biochem. Biophys. Res. Commun.* **217**, 640–648.

Kuchan, M. J. and Frangos, J. A. (1994) Role of calcium and calmodulin in flow induced NO production in endothelial cells. *Am. J. Physiol.* **266**, C628–C636.

Kufahl, R. H. and Saha, S. (1990) A theoretical model for stress-generated fluid-flow in the canaliculi lacunae network in bone tissue. *J. Biomech.* **23**, 171–180.

Lanyon, L. E. (1987) Functional strain in bone tissue as an objective and controlling stimulus for adaptive bone remodelling. *J. Biomech.* **20**, 1083–1093.

Lanyon, L. E. (1992) The success and failure of the adaptive response to functional load-bearing in averting bone fracture. *Bone* **13**, S17–S21.

Lanyon, L. E., Goodship, A. E., Pye, C. J. and MacFie, J. H. (1982) Mechanically adaptive bone remodelling. *J. Biomech.* **15**, 141–145.

Löwik, C. W. G. M., Nibbering, P. H., van de Ruit, M. and Papapoulos, S. E. (1994) Inducible production of nitric oxide in osteoblast-like cells and in fetal mouse bone explant is associated with suppression of osteoclastic bone resorption. *J. Clin. Invest.* **93**, 1465–1472.

Mayer, B., Moser, R., Gleispach, H. and Kukovetz, W. R. (1986) Possible inhibitory function of endogenous 15-hydroperoxyeicosatetraenoic acid on prostacyclin formation in bovine aortic endothelial cells. *Biochim. Biophys. Acta.* **875**, 641–653.

Murray, D. W. and Rushton, N. (1990) Effect of strain on bone cell prostaglandin E_2 release: a new experimetal method. *Calcif. Tiss. Int.* **47**, 35–39.

Nudel, U., Zakut, R., Shani, M., Neuman, S., Levy, Z. and Yaffe, D. (1983) Nucleotide sequence of the rat cytoplasmic β-actin gene. *Nucl. Acids Res.* **11**, 1759–1771.

Nunokawa, Y., Ishida, N. and Tanaka, S. (1993) Cloning of inducible NO synthase in rat vascular smooth muscle cells. *Biochem. Biophys. Res. Commun.* **191**, 89–94.

Olesen, S. P., Clapham, D. E. and Davies, P. F. (1988) Hemodynamic shear-stress activates a K^+ current in vascular endothelial cells. *Nature* **331**, 168–170.

Pead, M. J. and Lanyon, L. E. (1989) Indomethacin modulation of load-related stimulation of new bone formation *in vivo*. *Calcif. Tiss. Int.* **45**, 34–40.

Pead, M. J., Suswillo, R., Skerry, T. M., Vedi, S. and Lanyon, L. E. (1988) Increased ^3H uridine levels in osteocytes following a single short period of dynamic bone loading *in vivo*. *Calcif. Tiss. Int.* **43**, 92–96.

Pitsillides, A. A., Rawlinson, S. C. F., Suswillo, R. F. L. and Lanyon, L. E. (1995a) Nitric oxide production is stimulated by mechanical loading. *Bone* **16**, 682.

Pitsillides, A. A., Rawlinson, S. C. F., Suswillo, R. F. L., Bourrin, S., Zaman, G. and Lanyon, L. E. (1995b) Mechanical strain-induced NO production by bone cells: a possible role in adaptive bone (re)modeling? *FASEB J.* **9**, 1614–1622.

Pitsillides, A. A., Rawlinson, S. C. F., Suswillo, R. F. L., Zaman, G., Nijweide, P. J. and Lanyon, L. E. (1995c) Mechanical strain-induced NO production by osteoblasts and osteocytes. *J. Bone Min. Res.* **10**, S217.

Pitsillides, A. A., Rawlinson, S. C. F., Suswillo, R. F. L. *et al.* (1997) A putative role for osteocyte eNOS derived NO in adaptive bone (re)modelling: an extension to an endothelial paradigm. *Int. J. Exp. Pathol.* **77**, A40.

Pollack, S. R., Petrov, N., Salzstein, R., Brankov, G. and Blagoeva, R. (1984) An anatomical model for streaming potentials in osteons. *J. Biomech.* **17**, 627–636.

Ralston, S. H., Todd, D., Helfrich, M., Benjamin, N. and Grabowski, P. S. (1994) Human osteoblast-like cells produce nitric oxide and express inducible nitric oxide synthase. *Endocrinology* **135**, 330–336.

Rawlinson, S. C. F., El-Haj, A. J., Minter, S. L. J., Tavares, I. A., Bennett, A. and Lanyon, L. E. (1991) Loading related increases in prostaglandin production in cores of adult canine cancellous bone *in vitro*: a role for prostacyclin in adaptive bone remodelling? *J. Bone Min. Res.* **6**, 1345–1351.

Rawlinson, S. C. F., Mohan, S., Baylink, D. J. and Lanyon, L. E. (1993) Exogenous prostacyclin, but not prostaglandin E_2, produces similar responses in both G6PD activity and RNA production as mechanical loading, and increases IGF-II release, in adult cancellous bone in culture. *Calcif. Tiss. Int.* **53**, 324–329.

Rawlinson, S. C. F., Mosley, J. R., Suswillo, R. F. L., Pitsillides, A. A. and Lanyon, L. E. (1995) Calvarial and limb bone cells in organ and monolayer culture do not show the same early responses to dynamic mechanical strain. *J. Bone Min. Res.* **10**, 1225–1232.

Rawlinson, S. C. F., Pitsillides, A. A. and Lanyon, L. E. (1996) Involvement of different ion channels in osteoblasts' and osteocytes' early responses to mechanical strain. *Bone* **19**, 609–614.

Reich, K. M. and Frangos, J. A. (1991) Effect of flow on prostaglandin-E_2 and inosital triphosphate levels in osteoblasts. *Am. J. Physiol.* **261**, C428–C432.

Riancho, J. A., Salas, E., Zarrabeitia, M. T. *et al.* (1995) Expression and functional role of nitric oxide synthase in osteoblast-like cells. *J. Bone Min. Res.* **10**, 439–446.

Roer, R. D. and Dillaman, R. M. (1990) Bone-growth and calcium balance during simulated weightlessness in the rat. *J. Appl. Physiol.* **68**, 13–20.

Roux, W. (1881) In *Gesammelte abhandlungen aber die entwicklungsmechanik der organismen engelmenn*. Leipzig, 1885 (cited by Rosler, 1981).

Rubin, C. T. and Lanyon, L. E. (1984a) Dynamic strain similarity in vertebrates – an alternative to allometric limb bone scaling. *J. Theor Biol.* **107**, 321–327.

Rubin, C. T. and Lanyon, L. E. (1984b) Regulation of bone formation by applied dynamic loads. *J. Bone Joint Surg.* **66A**, 397–402.

Salvemini, D., Misko, T. P., Masferrer, J. L., Seibert, K., Currie, M. G. and Needleman, P. (1993) Nitric oxide activated cyclooxygenase enzymes. *Proc. Natl. Acad. Sci., USA.* **90**, 7240–7244.

Salvemini, D., Currie, M. G. and Mollace, V. (1996) Nitric oxide-mediated cyclooxygenase activation – a key event in antiplatelet effect of nitrovasodilators. *J. Clin. Invest.* **97**, 2562–2568.

Salzstein R. A. and Pollack, S. R. (1987) Electromechanical potentials in cortical bone: II. Experimental analysis. *J. Biomech.* **20**, 271–280.

Salzstein, R. A., Pollack, S. R., Mak, A. F. T. and Petrov, N. (1987) Electromechanical potentials in cortical bone: I. A continuum approach. *J. Biomech.* **20**, 261–270.

Shrör, K., Woditsch, I., Strobach, H. and Schröder, H. (1991) Interactions between nitric oxide and prostacyclin in myocardial ischemia and endothelial cell cultures. *Basic Res. Cardiol.* **86**, 117–125.

Skerry, T. M., Bitensky, L., Chayen, J. and Lanyon, L. E. (1989) Early strain-related changes in enzyme activity in osteocytes following bone loading *in vivo*. *J. Bone Min. Res.* **4**, 783–788.

Smith, E. L. and Gilligan, C. (1970) Mechanical forces and bone. *J. Bone Min. Res.* **6**, 139–173.

Takeda, K., Schini, V. and Stoeckel, H. (1987) Voltage-activated potassium, but not calcium, currents in cultured bovine aortic endothelial cells. *Pflugers Arch.: Eur. J. Physiol.* **410**, 385–393.

Tang, L. Y., Cullen, D. M., Yee, J. A., Jee, W. S. S. and Kimmel, D. B. (1997) Prostaglandin E(2) increases the skeletal response to mechanical loading. *J. Bone Min. Res.* **12**, 276–282.

Turner, C. H., Forwood, M. R. and Otter, M. W. (1994) Mechanotransduction in bone: do bone cells act as sensors of fluid-flow? *FASEB J.* **8**, 875–878.

Turner, C. H., Takano, Y., Owan, I. and Murrell, G. A. C. (1996) Nitric oxide inhibitor L-NAME- suppresses mechanically induced bone formation in rats. *Am. J. Physiol.* **270**, E634–E639.

van der Plaas, A. and Nijweide, P. J. (1992) Isolation and purification of osteocytes. *J. Bone Min. Res.* **7**, 389–396.

Vane, J. R., Mitchell, J. A., Appleton, I. *et al.* (1994) Inducible isoforms of cycloxygenase and nitric-oxide synthase in inflammation. *Proc. Natl. Acad. Sci., USA.* **91**, 2046–2050.

Weinbaum, S., Cowin, S. C. and Zeng, Y. (1994) A model for the excitation of osteocytes by mechanical load-induced fluid shear stresses. *J. Biomech.* **27**, 339–360.

Wilson, R. I., Yanovsky, J., Godecke, A., Stevens, D. R., Schrader, J. and Haas, H. L. (1997) Endothelial nitric oxide synthase and LTP. *Nature* **386**, 338.

Wimalawansa, S. J., de Marco, G., Gangula, P. and Yallampalli, C. (1996) Nitric oxide donor alleviates ovariectomy-induced bone loss. *Bone* **18**, 301–304.

Wolff, J. (1892) *Das Gesetz der Transformation der Knochen*. Hirschwald, Berlin. In translation: by Maguet, P. and Furlong, R. (1986) *The Law of Bone Remodelling*. Springer-Verlag, Berlin.

Yeh, C. K. and Rodan, G. A. (1984) Tensile forces enhance prostaglandin E synthesis in osteoblastic cells grown on collagen ribbons. *Calcif. Tiss. Int.* **36**, S67–S71.

Zaman, G., Suswillo, R. F. L., Cheng, M. Z., Tavares, I. A. and Lanyon, L. E. (1997) Early responses to dynamic strain change and prostaglandins in bone-derived cells in culture. *J. Bone Min. Res.* **12**, 769–777.

16

The response of bone and bone cells to mechanical stimulation

TIM J. CHAMBERS, JADE W. M. CHOW, SIMON FOX,
RON L. HOWARD, CHRISTOPHER. J. JAGGER, JENNY
M. LEAN, FREDERICK T. MITCHELL and ROLF SMALT

16.1 Introduction

The adaptability of the skeleton to mechanical loads is well established. The shape of bones is determined by the genetic programme, upon which is superimposed adaption to the mechanical environment. The distinct contribution of these two influences is most clearly seen in limb bones, in which mechanical usage causes a substantial change in shape and an increase in the quantity of bone compared with that determined genetically (Lanyon, 1980). Such mechanically adapted bones show a remarkably consistent strain response to mechanical usage: peak strains of 2000–3000 $\mu\varepsilon$ are observed over the cortical surface of bones in a wide variety of species during physiological activity (Rubin and Lanyon, 1984a).

The mechanisms by which mechanical forces regulate the structure and quantity of bone are poorly understood, but understanding them could provide opportunities to mimic or amplify the responses of bone to mechanical stimuli as a strategy to prevent fractures in diseases such as osteoporosis. Several approaches have been used to analyse this responsiveness. These include overload of the radius by ulnar osteotomy, external force application through implanted pins, external force application using four-point bending, and cyclic ulnar compression. It has been found that strains of physiological magnitude are sufficient to induce new bone formation in both avian and mammalian species (Rubin and Lanyon, 1984b; Turner *et al.*, 1991; Chow, Jagger and Chambers, 1993; Torrence *et al.*, 1994). It is believed that this osteogenic response to strains of only physiological magnitude occurs because the distribution of strains engendered by the mechanical stimulus within the bone are different from those to which it is accustomed (Lanyon, 1984).

It has been suggested that the cells best placed to sense the magnitude and distribution of strains are osteocytes. These cells form an interconnecting three-dimensional network throughout the matrix, where they are strategically placed both to respond to changes in strain and to disseminate information to surface cells of the osteoblastic lineage via a dense network of canalicular processes and communicating gap junctions.

169

16.2 Response of bone to mechanical stimulus

The experimental model we have developed to study the response of bone to mechanical stimulation uses pins, inserted through the 7th and 9th caudal vertebrae of rats, to exert a compressive load on the 8th vertebra (Figure 16.1). A single, 10 min application of external loading, sufficient to cause strains within the physiological range, is followed by a substantial osteogenic response over the ensuing 7–10 days (Chow *et al.*, 1993). An osteogenic response to strains of only physiological intensity is observed in other experimental models also. Osteogenesis occurs through the sensation not of supraphysiological strains but of strains imposed in an unaccustomed direction or distribution. This is believed to represent the mechanism by which bones adapt their structure to match changes in the mechanical environment. Therefore, while the forces to which the rat tail vertebra is normally exposed are unknown, when the bone is exposed to strains known to be experienced by other bones during mechanical usage, osteogenesis occurs. This is presumably analagous to the process whereby mechanical forces modify the shape of bones from that which would develop in their absence (e.g. Lanyon, 1980).

16.3 Molecular basis

The model system described above provides an opportunity to analyse the sequence of events after a temporally defined stimulus that leads to the initiation of bone formation. We have assessed mRNA expression of an early response gene c-*fos* (Lean *et al.*, 1996), and genes for IGF-I, collagen and osteocalcin by *in situ* hybridization (Lean *et al.*, 1995). We have found that there is early expression of c-*fos* in osteocytes and on bone surfaces such that, while we have never detected c-*fos* in the cortex of non-loaded bones, 20–30% of osteocytes in mechanically stimulated vertebrae strongly express c-*fos* within 30 min of loading (Figure 16.2). Expression is again undetectable by 6 h. Osteocytes also express IGF-I shortly after mechanical stimulation, but induction of expression is more gradual, reaches a peak after 6 h and persists for 1–2 days. Subsequently, IGF-I mRNA is detected on bone surfaces, soon followed by expression of matrix proteins, osteocalcin and collagen 1. Matrix protein synthesis is maximal 72 h after a mechanical stimulus

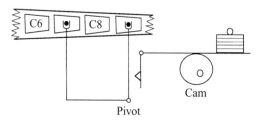

Figure 16.1 Diagram of apparatus used to impose dynamic strains on rat 8th caudal vertebrae. C6 is used as an internal control.

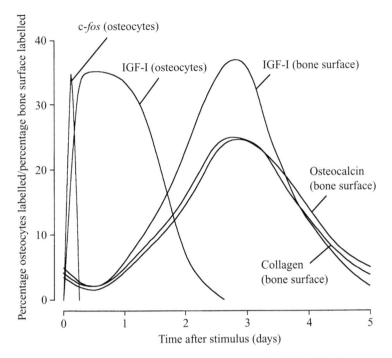

Figure 16.2 Diagrammatic representation of the temporal relationship of gene expression in osteocytes and on bone surfaces after mechanical stimulation of 8th caudal vertebrae, as assessed from *in situ* hybridization experiments.

and returns towards basal levels 5 days after loading. These increases in gene expression are accompanied by the induction of increased numbers of osteoblasts on bone surfaces and increases in mineralizing surfaces, as measured through the use of double fluorochrome labels.

Induction of expression of c-*fos* and IGF-I shortly after mechanical stimulation has also been detected by Northern blot analysis of extracts of bone in the four-point bending model of mechanical stimulation (Raab-Cullen *et al.*, 1994), and c-*fos* has been found by RT-PCR in extracts from the cortex of externally loaded rat ulna (Mason, Hillam and Skerry, 1996). Early expression of RNA is osteocytes, 2–3 days before an osteogenic response is detected on bone surfaces, strongly implicates osteocytes in the early transduction of mechanical strain signals.

It would clearly be of great interest to identify the mechanisms by which c-*fos* and the gene for IGF-I are induced in osteocytes and the events subsequent to their expression that eventuate in bone formation. The available evidence suggests that distinct signalling systems are responsible for the expression of these genes. Therefore, expression of both genes is independent of protein synthesis, suggesting that expression of one protein does not account for expression of the other (Lean *et al.*, 1996). Moreover, the spatial distribution of osteocytes expressing c-*fos* differs from that of the IGF-I gene: IGF-I gene is expressed primarily in osteocytes in the central parts of the mid-diaphysis, while osteocytes expressing c-*fos* are evenly distributed from periosteum to endosteum in the mid-diaphysis. Bone lining cells and cortical vascular channels also show very early expression of c-*fos* but not of the gene for IGF-I. The genes also differ in their sensitivity to inhibitors of prostaglandin synthesis (see below).

We chose to assess expression of IGF-I after mechanical stimulation because it is one of the most abundant growth factors secreted by bone cells, it induces proliferation and differentiation in osteoblastic cells and it has anabolic actions *in vivo* (Lean *et al.*, 1995). The early expression of this growth factor in osteocytes is, therefore, consistent with a model whereby IGF-I diffuses along osteocytic canaliculi to bone surfaces where it might participate in the induction and/or regulation of bone formation.

16.4 The role of prostaglandins

IGF-I production in osteoblastic cells is stimulated by prostagandins (McCarthy *et al.*, 1991). Could prostaglandins be responsible for osteocytic IGF-I production? Certainly, there is a substantial body of evidence for a role for prostaglandins in the mechanical responsiveness of bone. For examples, an early response of osteoblastic cells to mechanical strain is partly dependent on prostaglandins (Yeh and Rodan, 1984); exogenous prostaglandins stimulate bone formation *in vivo* (Norrdin *et al.*, 1990) and bone nodule formation *in vitro* (Flanagan and Chambers, 1992) and indomethacin inhibits mechanically induced osteogenesis *in vivo* (Pead and Lanyon, 1989; Chow and Chambers, 1994). We found (Chow and Chambers 1994) that the induction of bone formation by mechanical stimulation in the 8th caudal vertebra was inhibited by the administration of a single dose of indomethacin 3 h before loading; the same dose given 6 h after loading had no effect. This is consistent with a role for prostaglandins early in the osteogenic response. We also found that osteocytic IGF-I gene expression was strongly suppressed, and c-*fos* expression was partially suppressed, by indomethacin (Lean *et al.*, 1996).

The requirement for prostaglandin synthesis at the time of mechanical stimulation suggests involvement of COX in the transduction of osteocytic IGF-I expression and other osteogenic signals. However, we also identified a distinct late phase of indomethacin sensitivity for the osteogenic process. Presumably, events in the brief loading period are likely to entrain complex and sequential interactions between bone cells, and one or more of these interactions may involve prostaglandin-dependent steps. For example, growth factors can stimulate prostaglandin production, and prostaglandins induce growth factor production, by osteoblastic cells. *In vivo*, heterotopic bone formation by growth factors present in demineralized bone implants is inhibited by indomethacin. Production of COX-2 is increased by prostaglandins and has been shown to be induced by mechanical stimulation of bone *in vivo* (Forwood, 1996; and our unpublished observations). Therefore, prostaglandins seem to be important not only during the immediate–

early response to loading, when osteocytic IGF-I is induced, but also in subsequent interactions between cells and growth factors, which are likely to be necessary for the formation of new bone.

16.5 NO and the osteogenic response

The different sensitivity of osteocytic IGF-I gene and c-*fos* expression to suppression by indomethacin implies the existence of a second signal mediating mechanical responsiveness in ostocytes. Mechanical stimulation has been found to induce G6PD activity in osteocytes (Skerry *et al.*, 1989). This enzyme is responsible for the generation of NADPH, which is a co-enzyme for NOS, among other enzymes. We, therefore, tested the possibility that NO production plays a role in the osteogenic response. We found that the competitive NOS inhibitor L-NMMA, given to rats 15 min before mechanical stimulation, completely inhibited the increase in bone formation induced by mechanical stimulation in rat vertebrae (Fox, Chambers and Chow, 1996). The same dose administered 6 h after loading had no effect. This suppression was prevented by the coadministration of L-arginine, the natural substrate of NOS, but not the inactive stereoisomer D-arginine. Bone formation in non-loaded vertebrae or tibiae were unaffected by these protocols. Turner *et al.* (1996) independently reported inhibition of bone formation by L-NAME in the four-point bending model of mehanical osteogenesis.

Administration of L-NMMA at the dosage we used inhibits NO production for 30–60 min. Therefore, in animals given L-NMMA 15 min before loading, NO synthesis would be inhibited for up to 45 min after loading. This suggests that cNOS, which has recently been detected in bone cells (Pitsillides *et al.*, 1995; Riancho *et al.*, 1995), is responsible for the loading response. Suppression of the osteogenic response by brief inhibition of NOS activity around the time of loading itself is not consitsent with a role for iNOS, for which the lag time for transcription is 2 h; in addition, whereas high concentrations of NO, as typically generated by iNOS, inhibit proliferation, the relatively small quantities likely to be produced in bone by cNOS stimulate osteoblast proliferation *in vitro* (Fox *et al.*, 1996).

NO has been shown to activate c-*fos* expression (Abate *et al.*, 1990). In unpublished experiments, we have found partial (approximately 50%) suppression of c-*fos* by L-NMMA, as indicated by Northern blot analysis of RNA extracted from the cortex of loaded vertebrae. Indomethacin causes a similar suppression.

Both the induction of bone formation and the increase in G6PD activity after mechanical stimulation are suppressed by indomethacin (El Haj *et al.*, 1990; Chow and Chambers, 1994). This raises the possibility that mechanically induced bone formation is dependent on NO production, which in turn is dependent on prostaglandin production. Alternatively, prostaglandin and NO might both be required for mechanically induced osteogenesis, but they might be generated independently of each other.

16.6 The role of mechanical strain

It would greatly facilitate an analysis of these signalling pathways to have access to a cell culture system in which responses that reflect those occurring during mechanical transduction *in vivo* could be studied *in vitro*. There is, however, dispute over the appropriate mechanical stimulus. Suggestions include cell deformation as a direct result of strain in the load-bearing matrix or strain-induced fluid flow through the lacuno-canalicular network of bone, which might act through the generation of streaming potentials (which develop when charged moieties flow over a surface) or wall-shear stress (Chapter 14).

Many experiments have shown that bone cells are sensitive to mechanical strain *in vitro*. Most such studies, though, have used systems known to or likely to expose the cells to very large strains. Therefore, cells in cultures on flexible membranes experience strains between 3 and 24%, in contrast to the strains of up to 3000 $\mu\varepsilon$ (0.3%) measured under physiological loading conditions. Many cell types are sensitive to strain at these very high levels, so it is uncertain whether the responses induced in bone cells reflect the mechanisms by which bone normally senses mechanical stimuli, or whether they reflect responses also observed in non-osseous cells, which are presumably mounted for other purposes. In fact, experiments reporting a response to physiological strain are rare. Murray and Rushton (1990) found prostaglandin production by osteoblastic cells at approximately 8000 $\mu\varepsilon$; Jones *et al.* (1991) noted calcium transients in cells exposed to physiological strain loads. However, very prolonged periods of stimulation (e.g. 5 h) were used compared with the duration of stimulus that is effective *in vivo* (minutes). Recently, strains of physiological magnitude exerted by 4-point bending of plastic culture substrates have been shown to induce prostaglandin and NO production by bone cells (Pitsillides *et al.*, 1995).

16.7 The role of fluid flow

As an alternative to strain, bone cells might detect mechanical signals through fluid flow. Mechanical loading of bone causes flow of interstitial fluid through the canalicular network. Experimental evidence has been obtained that interstitial fluid flow affects the rate of bone formation in rats (Turner, Forwood and Otter, 1994). Weinbaum, Cowin and Zeng (1994) have proposed that fluid flow through canaliculi provides the mechanism by which bone cells experience the very small strains measured in bone during mechanical stimulation. Such a mechanism implies that bone cells must be sensitive to fluid-flow-induced wall-shear stresses of about 8–30 dyne/cm^2, which have been predicted to result from normal mechanical usage and which are similar to those acting on vascular endothelial cells. Reich and Frangos (1991) have reported induction of osteoblastic prostaglandin production by fluid flow in this range. Klein-Nulend *et al* (1995) noted prostaglandin production by osteocytes subjected to wall-shear stress, and Frangos' group (Johnson, McAllister and Frangos, 1996) noted that a wall-shear stress of 6 dyne/cm^2 caused NO production continuously for 12 h (Chapter 14).

16.8 Mechanical strain, fluid flow, NO and prostaglandins

We have attempted to compare the ability of mechanical strain and fluid flow to induce NO and prostaglandin production in bone cells. To do this we developed an experimental model in which bone cells are exposed to measurable and physiological strains in the absence of significant levels of fluid flow, by incubating the cells on strips of polystyrene film (Figure 16.3). For fluid flow experiments, we adapted a model (the parallel plate flow chamber) commonly used in the assessment of endothelial cell responses. We could detect no induction of either prostaglandin or NO production by cyclic strains (1 Hz) up to 5000 $\mu\varepsilon$. In contrast, low levels of fluid flow induced rapid production of both agents. NO production was observed after an increase in fluid flow for only 5 s and continued for up to 20 min after stimulation. Production was rapidly induced by fluid flow in the range 1–48 dyne/cm^2 and was observed in all the osteoblastic populations used (calvarial and long bone osteoblastic cells, MC3T3-E1, UMR 106.01 and ROS 17/2.8) but not in fibroblasts. When viscosity was increased with methylcellulose, there was increased responsiveness, suggesting that fluid flow stimulates osteoblastic cells through wall-shear stress.

Since NO and prostaglandin production appear to be essential for mechanical responsiveness *in vivo*, the observation that even relatively large mechanical strains do not cause detectable production of these compounds *in vitro*, while fluid flow induces both in the same cell populations, suggests that fluid flow is more likely to be the stimulas acting directly on the bone cells *in vivo*. There are caveats, though. We did not test the responsiveness of osteocytes, considered to be the primary transducers of mechanical information, although it would be surprising if no

(a)

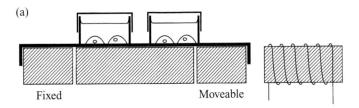

Fixed   Moveable

(b)

Inflow

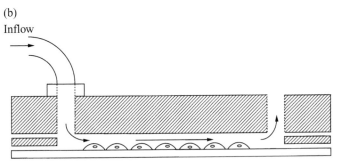

Figure 16.3 Experimental models used to test the effects of (a) mechanical strain and (b) the effects of fluid flow on bone cells *in vitro*.

osteocytic characteristics were expressed by cell populations of the same lineage, which can differentiate into undoubted osteocytes during bone nodule formation. For fluid flow at least, the particular responsiveness of osteocytes *in vivo* is explicable on the basis of their anatomical location rather than through some special characteristic not shared with other cells of the lineage. A second caveat is that the shear stresses to which bone cells are undoubtedly exposed during physiological usage have never been quantified. Nevertheless, fluid flow is a major determinant of endothelial cell behaviour, yet osteoblasts are even more sensitive to fluid flow.

16.9 Conclusions

The mechanisms by which detection of fluid flow by bone cells could be translated into information that allows bone to adapt its structure in a way appropriate for the mechanical environment is unknown. The remodelling of capillary beds by fluid flow during development suggests that information from fluid flow can be translated into morphogenetic decisions. While prostaglandin and NO production might both represent signals that directly regulate bone formation and resorption, it is equally possible that they, and other signals generated by fluid flow, are involved in the processing of mechanically generated information by bone cells. Whatever their role, our experiments suggest that fluid flow is the primary stimulus whereby bone cells respond to mechanical stimulation. If this is so, analysis of the effects of fluid flow on the behaviour of bone cells should provide insights into the processes whereby the skeleton adapts its structure to meet the challenges of the mechanical environment.

References

Abate, C., Patel, L., Rauscher III, F. J. and Curran, T. (1990) Redox regulation of *fos* and *jun* DNA-binding activity *in vitro*. *Science* **249**, 1157–1161.

Chow, J. W. M. and Chambers, T. J. (1994) Indomethacin has distinct early and late actions on bone formation induced by mechanical stimulation. *Am. J. Physiol.* **267**, E287–E292.

Chow, J. W. M., Jagger, C. J. and Chambers, T. J. (1993) Characterization of osteogenic response to mechanical stimulation in cancellous bone of rat caudal vertebrae. *Am. J. Physiol.* **265**, E340–E347.

El Haj, A. J., Minter, S. L., Rawlinson, S. C. F., Suswillo, R. and Lanyon, L. E. (1990) Cellular responses to mechanical loading *in vitro*. *J. Bone Min. Res.* **5**, 923–932.

Flanagan, A. M. and Chambers, T. J. (1992) Stimulation of bone nodule formation *in vitro* by prostaglandins E_1 and E_2. *Endocrinology* **130**, 443–448.

Forwood, M. R. (1996) Inducible cyclo-oxygenase (COX-2) mediates the induction of bone formation by mechanical loading *in vivo*. *J. Bone Min. Res.* **11**, 1688–1693.

Fox, S. W., Chambers, T. J. and Chow, J. W. M. (1996) Nitrix oxide is an early mediator of the increase in bone formation by mechanical stimulation. *Am. J. Physiol.* **270**, E955–E960.

Johnson, D. L., McAllister, T. N. and Frangos, J. A. (1996) Fluid-flow stimulates rapid and continuous release of nitric oxide in osteoblasts. *Am. J. Physiol.* **34**, E205–E208.

Jones, D. B., Nolte, H., Scholübbers, J. G., Turner, E. and Veltel, D. (1991) Biochemical signal transduction of mechanical strain in osteoblast-like cells. *Biomaterials* **12**, 101–110.

Klein-Nulend, J., van der Plas, A., Semeins, C. M. *et al.* (1995) Sensitivity of osteocytes to biomechanical stress *in vitro*. *FASEB J.* **9**, 441–445.

Lanyon, L. E. (1980) The influence of function on the development of bone curvature. An experimental study on the rat tibia. *J. Zool.* **192**, 457–466.

Lanyon, L. E. (1984) Functional strain as a determinant for bone remodelling. *Calcif. Tiss. Int.* **36**, S56–S61.

Lean, J. M., Jagger, C. J., Chambers, T. J. and Chow, J. W. M. (1995) Increased insulin-like growth factor I mRNA expression in rat osteocytes in response to mechanical stimulation. *Am. J. Physiol.* **268**, E318–E327.

Lean, J. M., Mackay, A. G., Chow, J. W. M and Chambers, T. J. (1996) Osteocytic expression of mRNA for c-*fos* and IGF-I: an immediate early gene response to an osteogenic stimulus. *Am. J. Physiol.* **270**, E937–E945.

Mason, D. J., Hillam, R. A. and Skerry, T. M. (1996) Constitutive *in vivo* mRNA expression by osteocytes of β-actin, osteocalcin, connexin-43, IGF-I, c-*fos* and c-*jun*, but not TNF-α nor tartrate-resistant acid phosphatase. *J. Bone Min. Res.* **11**, 350–357.

McCarthy, T. L., Centrella, M., Raisz, L. G. and Canalis, E. (1991) Prostaglandin E_2 stimulates insulin-like growth factor I synthesis in osteoblast-enriched cultures from fetal rat bone. *Endocrinology* **128**, 2895–2900.

Murray, D. W. and Rushton, N. (1990) The effect of strain on bone cell prostaglandin E_2 release: a new experimental method. *Calcif. Tiss. Int.* **47**, 35–39.

Norrdin, R. W., Jee, W. S. S. and High, W. B. (1990) Review: the role of prostaglandins in bone *in vivo*. *Prostaglandins, Leukotrienes and Essential Fatty Acids* **41**, 139–149.

Pead, M. J. and Lanyon, L. E. (1989) Indomethacin modulation of load-related stimulation of new bone formation *in vivo*. *Calcif. Tiss. Int.* **45**, 34–40.

Pitsillides, A. A., Rawlinson, S. C. F., Suswillo, R. F. L., Bourrin, S., Zaman, G. and Lanyon, L. E. (1995) Mechanical strain induced NO production by bone cells: a possible role in adaptive bone (re)modelling? *FASEB J.* **9**, 1614–1622.

Raab-Cullen, D. M., Thiede, M. A., Peterson, D. N., Kimmel, D. B. and Recker, R. R. (1994) Mechanical loading stimulates rapid changes in periosteal gene expression. *Calcif. Tiss. Int.* **55**, 473–478.

Reich, K. M. and Frangos, J. A. (1991) Effect of flow on prostaglandin E_2 and inositol triphosphate levels in osteoblasts. *Am. J. Physiol.* **261**, C428–C432.

Riancho, J. A., Salas, E., Zarrabeitia, M. T. *et al.* (1995) Expression and functional role of nitric oxide synthase in osteoblast-like cells. *J. Bone Min. Res.* **10**, 439–446.

Rubin, C. T. and Lanyon, L. E. (1984a) Dynamic strain similarity in vertebrates: an alternative to allometric limb bone scaling. *J. Theor. Biol.* **107**, 321–327.

Rubin, C. T. and Lanyon, L. E. (1984b) Regulation of bone formation by applied dynamic loads. *J. Bone Joint Surg.* **66A**, 397–402.

Skerry, T. M., Bitensky, L., Chayen, J. and Lanyon, L. E. (1989) Early strain-related changes in enzyme activity in osteocytes following bone loading *in vivo*. *J. Bone Min. Res.* **4**, 783–788.

Torrance, A. G., Mosley, J. R., Suswillo, R. F. and Lanyon, L. E. (1994) Noninvasive loading of the rat ulna *in vivo* induces a strain-related modeling response uncomplicated by trauma or periosteal pressure. *Calcif. Tiss. Int.* **54**, 241–247.

Turner, C. H., Akhter, M. P., Raab, D. M., Kimmel, D. B. and Recker, R. R. (1991) A noninvasive, *in vivo* model for studying strain adaptive bone modeling. *Bone* **12**, 73–79.

Turner, C. H., Forwood, M. R. and Otter, M. W. (1994) Mechanotransduction in bone: do bone cells act as sensors of fluid flow? *FASEB J.* **8**, 875–878.

Turner, C. H., Takano, Y., Owan, I. and Murrell, G. A. (1996) Nitric oxide inhibitor L-NAME suppresses mechanically induced bone formation in rats. *Am. J. Physiol.* **270**, E634–E639.

Weinbaum, S., Cowin, S. C. and Zeng, Y. (1994) A model for the excitation of osteocytes by mechanical loading-induced bone fluid shear stresses. *J. Biomech.* **27**, 339–360.

Yeh, C. K. and Rodan, G. A. (1984) Tensile forces enhance prostaglandin E synthesis in osteoblastic cells grown on collagen ribbons. *Calcif. Tiss. Int.* **36**, S67–S71.

17

Aseptic loosening of total hip prostheses

STEVEN A. CORBETT, MIKA V. J. HUKKANEN, SEAN P. F. HUGHES and JULIA M. POLAK

17.1 Introduction

Total hip replacement (THR) surgery has the potential to transform a patient's life by relieving the pain, disability or deformity that prompt the surgical intervention and in its ability to restore independent freedom. A major problem of such surgery is failure of the implant, necessitating revision surgery. In the UK, over 11 000 revision operations are currently performed each year. Aseptic loosening is the most common cause of early failure and, as it is estimated that by the year 2010 there will be 200 million patients worldwide with total hip replacements this represents a major clinical problem. Furthermore, revision surgery has a much lower success rate compared with primary replacement surgery; hence early prosthetic failure has significant patient, social and economic implications.

Aseptic loosening is a disease process in which the implant becomes loosened in the absence of infection. The expected life span of the prosthesis is considerably reduced, with the patient experiencing symptoms often similar to those of the original presenting complaint. Once established, the loosening may be visualized by X-ray analysis, where it is represented as areas of translucency compatible with bone resorption. Unfortunately, the initial sensitivity associated with standard X-ray techniques is limited, hence the diagnosis may only become apparent some time after the onset of the loosening process. However, more sophisticated techniques of assessment, such as radiostereometric analysis (RSA), have demonstrated that the prosthetic migration secondary to loosening may be observed within 2 years of the original operation. It is possible that the process of bone resorption at the bone–prosthesis interface begins even earlier.

Much research interest has focused on the interrelationships between the implant and host tissue response at a cellular level in an attempt to characterize the underlying pathogenesis of aseptic loosening. While the exact mechanism remains to be defined, increasing evidence indicates that cyclical mechanical loading, production of wear particles (Santavirta *et al.*, 1990; Schmalzried *et al.*, 1992) and the ensuing adverse tissue response to the wear particles (Murray and Rushton, 1990; Amstutz *et al.* 1992; Jiranek *et al.*, 1993) are all important

178

contributors to the aggressive local osteolysis and linear bone resorption at the bone–prosthesis interface. It is considered that the resultant cortical bone loss is caused by activation and release of a cascade of cell mediators by macrophages and other cells capable of phagocytosis of the prosthetic particulate debris.

17.2 Pseudomembrane

One of the characteristic features of the loosened prosthesis is the formation of an interface membrane with a pseudosynovial lining layer facing the prosthesis surface. Studies have shown the membrane to be characterized by the presence of macrophages and frequent giant cells, compatible with a chronic inflammatory reaction, while epipolarized light microscopy has shown that many of the cells are laden with wear debris. There is, however, considerable heterogeneity of tissue cell type, with a range of leukocyte presence, variability of macrophage expression and a small population of granulocytes and lymphocytes (Perry *et al.*, 1995). The membrane has been suggested to have three different histological patterns (Boynton *et al.*, 1995):

Type 1: mostly fibrous tissue with cells and macrophages widely scattered through the membrane
Type 2: fibrous membrane with a significant number of T cells, macrophages and foreign-body giant cells and well-defined foreign body granulomas
Type 3: diffusely scattered T cells, ill-defined granulomas, 'foamy' macrophages and fewer foreign-body giant cells than in Type 2.

Such distinction, however, may be difficult, as within the same patient the pseudomembrane may not be uniform, with different regions having different cellular characteristics. As THRs may be cemented or uncemented, it might be expected that there would be a difference between the ensuing membranes. It has been shown that cementless membranes contained more metal debris and cemented membranes more foreign-body giant cells (Kim *et al.*, 1993). While the histological differences between both membranes are obviously important, the most significant aspect is the ability of the membranes to release bioactive products that might induce bone resorption and cause aseptic loosening. In the same study, both membrane origins were shown to cause significant elevation of gelatinase, collagenase, the arachidonic metabolite PGE_2 and IL-1, thereby demonstrating the potential for inducing bone resorption.

17.3 Wear debris

Wear debris has been shown to have a variety of origins: from the metallic implant components (such as chrome–cobalt and titanium), from the acetabular component (polyethylene) and from any cement mantle present (e.g. polymethylmethacrylate). While there are certain critical factors, such as particle size and shape, that appear necessary in determining the resultant activity in the pseudomembrane, there is evidence that each particulate origin may have a role in the resultant disease process.

A common denominator for all debris activity appears to be the requirement for macrophage engulfment before bone resorption may occur. Whether the recruited macrophages then cause independent bone resorption by direct action or via a bone cell intermediary is subject to debate. It has been reported that macrophages appear to be the cells primarily responsible for bone loss in osteolytic lesions, rather than acting as cells producing inflammatory mediators that could activate osteoclasts (Kadoya *et al.*, 1996). However, there is considerable evidence that the macrophages do, in fact, cause osteoblast–osteoclast activation via cellular messengers. For example, it has been suggested that the interaction between macrophages and polymethylmethacrylate particles formed secondary to mechanical failure causes TNFα release. This subsequently provokes the release of GM-CSF, IL-6 and PGE$_2$ from osteoblasts, thereby causing further macrophage and osteoclast recruitment (Horowitz and Purdon, 1995; Pollice, Silverton and Horowitz, 1995).

17.4 Cytokines and NO

A number of cytokines and inflammatory mediators are expressed in interface membranes and found in synovial fluid. IL-1, TNFα and PGE$_2$ have all been strongly implicated in the induction and maintenance of bone resorption and demonstrated to be present in the pseudomembrane (Sedel *et al.*, 1992; Jiranek *et al.*, 1993; Al Saffar and Revell, 1994; Chiba *et al.*, 1994; Konttinen *et al.*, 1996). Cell culture experiments have confirmed the ability of isolated macrophages and pseudomembrane-derived cells to secrete IL-1, TNFα and PGE$_2$ and to stimulate bone resorption as a result of wear particle stimulation (Murray and Rushton, 1990; Westacott *et al.*, 1992; Hukkanen *et al.*, 1995; Algan, Purdon and Horowitz, 1996). It is recognized that these proinflammatory cytokines may induce the expression of iNOS to produce large quantities of NO. Therefore, the potential exists for NO to play a role in aseptic loosening. In addition, iNOS is involved in the modulation of the activity of other key metabolic enzymes such as COX-2; hence the presence of PGE$_2$ may also relate to iNOS activity.

Although NO is by definition a free radical, it is not particularly reactive or toxic at low levels because of its removal by reaction with haemoglobin. However its toxicity is much increased by its reaction with the superoxide anion to form peroxynitrite (Beckman *et al.*, 1994; Stamler, 1994; Buttery *et al.*, 1995). Peroxynitrite is known to cause oxidation of cell membrane lipids and DNA bases, thus contributing to cell death. NO can inactivate superoxide dismutase, leading to increased accumulation of superoxide anion, which itself can stimulate bone resorption, and also interfere with the glutathione–glutathione peroxidase system; this results in increased production of hydrogen peroxide, a reactive oxygen species able to activate bone resorption (Garrett *et al.*, 1990; Bax *et al.*, 1992). These NO-derived free radicals, therefore, may potentially be involved in aseptic loosening.

17.5 iNOS and COX-2 in aseptic loosening

In a recent study, we investigated whether the expression of iNOS and COX-2 are stimulated in periprosthetic macrophages and whether peroxynitrite-induced nitro-sylation can be detected in patients with failed total hip arthroplasties. This would provide a mechanism for wear particle- and cytokine-induced aggravation of local inflammation, bone resorption and prostanoid-induced pain characteristic of failed total hip arthroplasty. The results of our experiments provide evidence that iNOS and COX-2 proteins and their enzyme activities are present in the interface membranes and that CD68[+] macrophages are the major inflammatory cell population expressing immunoreactivity for iNOS, nitrotyrosine and COX-2 (Hukkanen *et al.*, 1997).

Our study demonstrated that prosthetic wear particles phagocytosed by macrophages found in the interface membrane are likely to contribute to the induction of iNOS by human macrophages. Calcium-independent iNOS enzymatic activity was found to be present in such tissues, providing evidence that NO is produced locally. Further evidence of local NO (and superoxide) production was provided by localization of nitrotyrosine, a marker of peroxynitrite-induced protein damage, in the interface membrane. Nitrotyrosine was found in cells immunoreactive for iNOS but also in others, suggesting both autocrine and paracrine effects of NO. Significant correlation between iNOS and COX-2 tissue distribution was noted and double immunolabelling of the proteins was used to show that both iNOS and COX-2 were found in the same cells, these being mainly CD68[+] macrophages. Therefore, it is very likely that phagocytosis of wear particles by macrophages will induce the synthesis of NO, with subsequent contribution to the induction of COX-2 mRNA, protein and enzymatic activity.

Our previous studies have shown that iNOS activity induced by IL-1, TNFα and IFNγ and high-output NO production result in inhibition of osteoblast proliferation, alkaline phosphatase activity and osteocalcin synthesis, which are markers of osteoblast maturation (Hukkanen *et al.*, 1995). This NO production is also involved in induction of apoptosis in osteoblast cultures (Hughes *et al.*, 1995; see also Chapter 10). However low output production of NO by the constitutive isoforms can exert beneficial effects on bone cell function. Recent work has suggested that both fluid sheer stress and mechanical strain may induce rapid and transient NO production by osteoblasts and osteocytes (Frangos and Johnson, 1995; Pitsillides *et al.*, 1995). Mechanical strain-induced new bone formation (Lanyon *et al.*, 1982) has now been shown to be largely mediated by a NO-dependent mechanism, as there is no new bone formation when prototypic NOS inhibitors are administered prior to the strain stimuli (Fox, Chambers and Chow, 1996; Turner *et al.*, 1996). Also, prostanoid production appears to have significant importance during the early stages of new bone formation and its adaptation to the mechanical strain (Chapter 15). Recently it has been demonstrated that physiological levels of mechanical strain induce nitrite production within minutes of the application of the strain (Chapter 15; Pitsillides *et al.*,

1997). This rapid NO production implies the presence of a constitutive isoform of NOS within the bone cells, and our recent studies have indeed shown the presence of the eNOS isoform in osteocytes and osteoblasts (Fernandez de Marticorena *et al.*, 1998).

17.6 Proposed model

It is possible to speculate from these findings that low level NO production by the eNOS isoform may be of central importance for the bone–implant bonding of the prostheses. Cyclical mechanical loading and micromovement of the prosthesis may activate the sheer stress element in the eNOS gene, resulting in low level NO production and maintenance of the bone–implant bond by continuous adaptation of the surrounding bone. However, when repetitive and excessive prosthetic loading occurs, with subsequent wear particle production, this leads to activation of inflammatory phagocytic cells, production of proinflammatory cytokines such as IL-1 and TNFα and the induction of iNOS and COX-2, with high output synthesis of NO, peroxynitrite and prostanoids. This would be detrimental to new bone growth and would accelerate the resorption and invasion by connective periprosthetic soft tissue, leading finally to aseptic loosening of the prosthesis.

17.7 Future development

According to the model described here, pharmacological suppression of the iNOS and COX-2 isoforms would be beneficial for the homeostasis of periprosthetic cancellous bone and would at least partially restore the adaptive nature of both the osteocytes and osteoblasts. It is interesting to note that addition of indomethacin, structurally unrelated NSAIDs, or corticosteroids to bone-cement membrane cultures has been shown to alter the process of bone resorption in the vicinity of cemented joint implants (Ohlin and Lerner, 1993). The anti-inflammatory, analgesic and anti-pyretic effects of NSAIDs are all thought to result from their ability to inhibit COX-2 enzyme activity and subsequent prostanoid production. Unfortunately, the current generation of NSAIDs also interfere with COX-1 activity, resulting in significant sequelae, such as ulceration. However, the newer specific inhibitors of COX-2, currently used for experimental purposes, may prove more beneficial. At the moment, there are no specific drugs for clinical use that can specifically suppress iNOS activity. However, many steroids are able to inhibit the synthesis of iNOS protein. Specific inhibition of iNOS protein expression or enzyme activity without interfering with the constitutive isoform of NOS might prove to be a useful means of suppressing the chronic inflammation associated with aseptic loosening.

In conclusion, there is evidence that the induction mechanisms for both iNOS and COX-2 are present and functioning in periprosthetic interface tissue from patients with failed total hip arthroplasty and these molecules may account for the aseptic loosening process.

References

Algan, S. M., Purdon, M. and Horowitz, S. M. (1996) Role of tumor necrosis factor alpha in particulate-induced bone resorption. *J. Orthop. Res.* **14**, 30–35.

Al Saffar, N. and Revell, P. A. (1994) Interleukin-1 production by activated macrophages surrounding loosened orthopaedic implants: a potential role in osteolysis. *Br. J. Rheumatol.* **33**, 309–316.

Amstutz, H. C., Campbell, P., Kossovsky, N. and Clarke, I. C. (1992) Mechanism and clinical significance of wear debris induced osteolysis. *Clin. Orthop.* **276**, 7–18.

Bax, B. E., Alam, A. S. M. T., Banerji, B. *et al.* (1992) Stimulation of osteoclastic bone resorption by hydrogen peroxidase. *Biochem. Biophys. Res. Commun.* **183**, 1153–1158.

Beckman, J. S., Chen, J., Crow, J. P. and Ye, Y. Z. (1994) Reactions of nitric oxide, superoxide and peroxynitrite with superoxide dismutase in neurodegeneration. In Seil FJ, ed. *Progress in Brain Research*, Vol. 103 (ed. F. J. Seil), pp. 371–380. Elsevier Science BV, Amsterdam.

Boynton, E. L., Henry, M., Morton, J. and Waddell, J. P. (1995) The inflammatory response to particulate wear debris in total hip arthroplasty. *Can. J. Surg.* **36**, 507–515.

Buttery, L. D. K., Hukkanen, M. V. J., O'Donnell, A., Polak, J. M. and Hughes, F. J. (1995) Nitric oxide dependent and independent induction of prostaglandin synthesis in osteoblasts. *Bone* **17**, 560.

Chiba, J., Rubash. H. E., Kim, K. J. and Iwaki, Y. (1994) The characterization of cytokines in the interface tissue obtained from failed cementless total hip arthroplasty with and without femoral osteolysis. *Clin. Orthop.* **300**, 304–312.

Fernandez de Marticorena, I., Platts, L. A. M., O'Shaughnessy, M., Chacon, M. R., Hukkanen, M. and Polak, J. M. (1998) Endothelial nitric oxide synthase (eNOS) is highly expressed during bone development and remodelling. *J. Pathol.*, in press.

Fox, S. W., Chambers, T. J. and Chow, J. W. M. (1996) Nitric oxide is an early mediator of the increase in bone formation by mechanical stimulation. *Am. J. Physiol.* **270**, E955–E960.

Frangos, J. A. and Johnson, D. L. (1995) Rapid flow-induced production of nitric oxide in osteoblasts. *Endothelium* **3**(Suppl.), S8.

Garrett, I. R., Boyce, B. F., Oreffo, R. O. C., Bonewald, L., Poser, J. and Mundy, G. R. (1990) Oxygen-derived free radicals stimulate osteoclastic bone resorption in rodent bone *in vitro* and *in vivo*. *J. Clin. Invest.* **85**, 632–639.

Horowitz, S. M. and Purdon, M. A. (1995) Mechanisms of cellular recruitment in aseptic loosening of prosthetic implants. *Calcif. Tiss. Int.* **57**, 301–305.

Hughes, F. J., Ghazi, R., Hukkanen, M., Buttery, L. and Polak, J. M. (1995) Cytokine-induced apoptosis in osteoblast cultures mediated by nitric oxide. *Bone* **17**, 565.

Hukkanen, M., Hughes, F. J., Buttery, L. D. K. *et al.* (1995) Cytokine-stimulated expression of nitric oxide synthase by mouse, rat and human osteoblast-like cells and its functional role in osteoblast metabolism. *Endocrinology* **136**, 5445–5453.

Hukkanen, M., Corbett, S. A., Batten, J. *et al.* (1997) Aseptic loosening of total hip replacement – macrophage expression of inducible nitric oxide synthase and cyclo-oxygenase-2, together with peroxynitrite formation as a possible mechanism for early prosthesis failure. *J. Bone Joint Surg.* **79B**, 467–474.

Jiranek, W. A., Machado, M., Jasty, M. *et al.* (1993) Production of cytokines around loosened cemented acetabular components: analysis with immunohistochemical techniques and *in situ* hybridization. *J. Bone Joint Surg.* **75A**, 863–879.

Kadoya, Y., Revell, P. A., Alsaffar, N., Kobayashi, A., Scott, G. and Freeman, M. A. R. (1996) Bone formation and bone resorption in failed total joint arthroplasties. Histomorphometric analysis with histochemical and immunohistochemical technique. *J. Orthop. Res.* **14**, 473–482.

Kim, K. J., Rubash, H. E., Wilson, S. C., D'Antonio, J. A. and McClain, E. J. (1993) A histological and biochemical comparison of the interface tissues in cementless and cemented hip prostheses. *Clin. Orthop.* **287**, 142–152.

Konttinen, Y. T., Kurvinen, H., Takagi, M. *et al.* (1996) IL-1 and collagenases around loose total hip prosthesis. *Clin. Exp. Rheumatol.* **14**, 255–262.

Lanyon, L. E., Goodship, A. E., Pye, C. J. and Macfie, J. H. (1982) Mechanically adaptive bone remodelling. *J. Biomech.* **15**, 141–145.

Murray, D. W. and Rushton, N. (1990) Macrophages stimulate bone resorption when they phagocytose particles. *J. Bone Joint Surg.* **72B**, 988–992.

Ohlin, A. and Lerner, U. H. (1993) Bone resorbing activity of different periprosthetic tissues in aseptic loosening of total hip arthroplasty. *Bone Min.* **20**, 67–78.

Perry, M. J., Mortuza, F. Y., Ponsford, F. M., Elson, C. J. and Atkins, R. M. (1995) Analysis of cell types and mediator production around loosened joint implants. *Br. J. Rheumatol.* **34**, 1127–1134.

Pitsillides, A. A., Rawlinson, S. C. F., Suswillo, R. F. L., Bourrin, S., Zaman, G. and Lanyon, L. E. (1995) Mechanical strain-induced NO production by bone cells: a possible role in adaptive bone (re)modeling? *FASEB J.* **9**, 1614–1622.

Pitsillides, A. A., Rawlinson, S. C. F., Suswillo, R. F. L. *et al.* (1997) A putative role for osteocyte endothelial nitric oxide synthase in adaptive bone (re)modelling. *Bone* **20**, 45–165.

Pollice, P. F., Silverton, S. F. and Horowitz, S. M. (1995) Polymethylmethacrylate-stimulated macrophages increase rat osteoclast precursor recruitment through their effect on osteoblasts *in vitro. J. Orthop. Res.* **13**, 325–334.

Santavirta, S., Konttinen, Y. T., Bergroth, V., Eskola, A., Tallroth, K. and Lindholm, T. S. (1990) Aggressive granulomatous lesions associated with hip arthroplasty: immuno-pathological studies. *J. Bone Joint Surg.*, **72A**, 252–258.

Schmalzried, T. P., Kwong, L. M., Jasty, M. *et al.* (1992) The mechanism of loosening of cemented acetabular components in total hip arthroplasty. Analysis of specimens retrieved at autopsy. *Clin. Orthop.* **274**, 60–78.

Sedel, L., Simeon, J., Meunier, A., Villette, J. M. and Launay, S. M. (1992) Prostaglandin E_2 level in tissue surrounding aseptic failed total hips. *Arch. Orthop. Trauma Surg.* **111**, 255–258.

Stamler, J. S. (1994) Redox signalling: nitrosylation and related target interactions of nitric oxide. *Cell* **78**, 931–936.

Turner, C. H., Takano, Y., Owan, I. and Murrell, G. A. C. (1996) Nitric oxide inhibitor L-NAME suppresses mechanically induced bone formation in rats. *Am. J. Physiol.* **270**, E634–E639.

Westacott, C. I., Taylor, G., Atkins, R. and Elson, C. (1992) Interleukin-1 alpha and beta production by cells isolated from membranes around aseptically loose total joint replacements. *Ann. Rheum. Dis.* **51**, 638–642.

Index